LAND of STONE

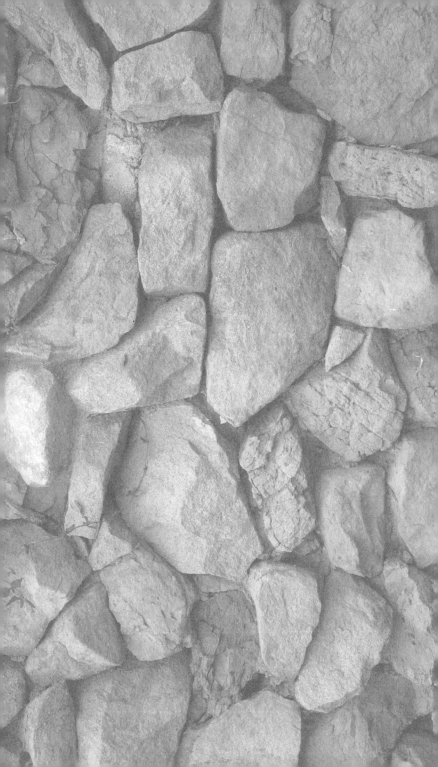

For the patients and staff of Seven and Eight South

The pencil lets you say what the mouth does not.
—A Rosedale Hospital patient

Contents

Preface

Land of Stone is a story about silence and kinship. For more than a decade, while continuing life as a practicing poet, I taught poetry writing to severely ill patients at Rosedale, a large psychiatric hospital outside of New York City. A man named Ben was a patient there in the mid-1980s. The story of how we worked together every week for two years, writing poems in near silence, goes against the grain of today's culture and now bears telling. To express one's experience slowly and indirectly is a simple human need, but as we zoom through the twenty-first century, telling each exquisite detail of our lives with no regard for pace or privacy, talk—a lot of it and fast—is everywhere.

Strikingly handsome Ben had been admitted to the hospital by his parents, who had lived through the Holocaust. He had been virtually silent for six years and sometimes was violent. When I met him on the ward, he often stood rigidly in one spot with an intense gaze or would burst into a big grin at apparently nothing.

Ben's family had moved back and forth between the

United States and Israel several times. As a boy, Ben excelled in his schoolwork, loved art, and won trophies as a runner. In junior high, he began to take drugs. He was expelled from high school for disrupting classes by talking too much. And then, for some reason, Ben stopped speaking. When he was first admitted to a psychiatric hospital at age twenty-four, he was so withdrawn that he was described as autistic. Ben had given up on words.

We met every week in near silence and alternated writing lines of poems. I wrote a line. Ben wrote a line. We played off of each other's lines like jazz players, improvising, doing solos, doing duets, never knowing what would come of it. With great hesitation, Ben chose to raise his voice—first on paper, then out loud. Eventually, he began to speak and became part of the talking world again.

Stories take a long time to tell. A few summers ago, I drove up the East Coast to Campobello Island. On a tour of Franklin Roosevelt's summer cottage, a guide showed me his small bedroom with a simple, single bed and window. There, FDR had been stricken with polio. The night he fell ill, a forest fire was raging on the island. I pictured him slowing down, his muscles weakening, his head full of fever, his neck stiffening— Roosevelt gazing out that window as fire consumed the island. I could not sleep that night, or the next. Years earlier, as a young girl, I had been paralyzed from polio. Although I recovered, it was an experience I was silent about.

As I watched Ben slowly begin to tell his story through metaphoric poems, I understood just how long it can take for a person to be ready to tell his story. For the two years we worked together, it did not occur to me that I, too, had a story. Although I was the hospital worker and Ben was the hospital patient, through our collaboration we both got better.

In fact, one day before I began work on the ward, a puzzling thing happened. I was on my way to the city branch of Rosedale for an interview, walking along the street toward the East River. It was cool, it was gorgeous, it was spring, and aside from being nervous about the interview, I was feeling fine and fit. Pausing before a tree planted in a small square of dirt set in the concrete sidewalk, I—with no warning—began to vomit uncontrollably.

A few years later, during a meeting with the psychiatrist who became my supervisor, I remembered that jarring day. As I told him the vomiting story, and as he questioned me, it dawned on me that I had been on my way to the very same hospital where, as a little girl, I had been a polio patient. Although it is hard to believe, until then I had failed to make the connection.

Since that first day when Ben and I began to write poems together, I had wondered what made our collaboration so magnetic. I wrote a line, Ben wrote a line—the phrase keeps recurring. Different from the dialogue that occurs in normal conversation, we offered each other intense attention, going back and forth, taking turns. As I wondered why I could collaborate with such a silent, stony character, I began to wonder about my own story as well as Ben's.

What made this particular collaboration so powerful? Ben seemed locked inside himself. He looked immobile, although physically he was fine. As a child paralyzed from polio, I was locked out of myself. Not to equate mental and physical paralysis, but we shared a parallel sense of immobility that propelled our collaboration forward.

Although Ben had been sporadically violent, it was his six-year silence that caused his parents to bring him to Rosedale Hospital. By then in his late twenties, Ben barely spoke when he first entered the ward. He could be found standing sphinxlike in the corridor staring at the wall or in the bathroom taking showers. In his first hospital interview, he expressed the view that he had only been in his mother's womb for three months before being born. Ben's psychiatrist told me that he never spoke spontaneously and would answer questions with one word or, at most, a brief phrase. Nevertheless, Ben agreed to meet with me. We wrote nearly two hundred poems in collaboration, and every week for two years, I wrote a line, he wrote a line.

Acknowledgments

To be welcomed into the community at the Rose-
dale Hospital was a rare privilege. Most of all, thanks
to the patients who lived on Seven South and Eight
South. Thanks especially to Ruth Obernbreit Glass,
Drs. Ann Appelbaum and Richard Munich, extraor-
dinary and generous teachers. Thanks to Drs. Frank
Yeomans, Mike Selzer, Eric Mendelsohn, Andy Lot-
terman, John Grimaldi, Monica Carsky, Bob Abrams,
Tsilia Glinberg, Priscilla Fischler, Diana Diamond,
Jonathan Kreiger, and the memory of Jane Doller.
Thanks to Synthia Pommiss, Norma Salmon, Robin
Weisman Gaines, and Juliet Goldsmith. To Dr. Ted
Shapiro, who first introduced me to Rosedale, thank
you. Thanks to Drs. Otto Kernberg and Bob Michels
for creating the fertile climate at Rosedale Hospital
that made this work possible.

I owe much to the late William Stafford—the wis-
dom in his poems and essays bolstered my own think-
ing about poetry and the hospital work.

Many thanks to the foundation funders who believed in the Poetry Project and kept it afloat: the van Ameringen Foundation, the Witter Bynner Foundation for Poetry, the Rockefeller Foundation, the Merck Family Fund, the Spunk Fund, the Public Welfare Foundation, Amy Cohen of the Scheuer Family Fund, and John and Lucia Mudd of the Lebensburger Foundation. Thanks also to Sid Knafel, Joyce and Mike Rappeport, Priscilla Ellsworth, and Emily Rechnitz. Thanks to the late Gerald Freund, a large-hearted supporter. Great gratitude to the Rockefeller Foundation's Bellagio Center for Artists and Scholars, where I worked on an early draft of *Land of Stone*.

Many thanks to the wonderful team at Wayne State University Press: Kristin Harpster Lawrence, Maya Rhodes, Renée Tambeau, and Sarah Murphy, as well as to the talented freelance copyeditor Kathleen Fields. To the supreme acquisitions editor Mollika Basu, who has been a pleasure to work with and know, a special thank you.

Enormous thanks to Didi Goldenhar, who has been an editor and friend without match through every stage of this book. Thank you Jonathan Matson, my treasured literary agent. To Dr. Paul Lippmann, many thanks for tutoring me in the subject of love and the human mind, a key ingredient in my hospital work. Thanks to friends who contributed to this book in numerous ways: Trudy Ames, Nina Ryan, Mary Bisbee-Beek, Londa Weisman, my sister and brother-in-law Maggi and Knute Walker, and special thanks to Joelle

ACKNOWLEDGMENTS

Sander for large doses of companionship, stimulating ideas, and jokes.

To my sons, David Chase and Matthew Chase-Daniel, teenagers when I began at Rosedale, you have always been my wisest teachers. And to my husband, Paul Graubard, to you, everything.

I Am a Stone
Ben Begins to Write

Summer is about to end. A light-colored car is caught in a traffic jam on the Brooklyn–Queens Expressway. The car has no air conditioner, the air is sticky and thick, and no one cracks a window. This is how I picture the scene. Mr. and Mrs. X are in the front seat, Ben and his older brother, Martin, in back. Except for an occasional futile horn and the whirr of traffic speeding the opposite way, there's no sound. No one complains, no one suggests rolling down a window, no one says a thing.

With no hint of trouble brewing, Ben grabs Martin by the shoulders and begins to shake him robotically and mercilessly. Mr. X swerves off the highway onto the wide right shoulder and pulls Ben off Martin. By then Martin is screaming bloody murder, Ben is saying nothing, Mrs. X is quiet, and Mr. X has halted the outburst. It is indescribably hot.

They pull back onto the road. Traffic inches along, then eventually picks up speed, and within half an hour the family arrives home. A few days later, Ben is sitting upright, his posture-perfect back straight, on the drab green living-room sofa, watching the weather report on TV. There's flooding in the Midwest; the Missouri has overflowed its banks. Towns are going underwater. Ben is watching aerial views of devastation. No amount of sandbagging, no amount of citizen effort, eases the disaster. The National Guard is rescuing people by helicopter. Ben, unmoving, is glued to the screen.

Arriving home from work, Mrs. X opens the front door, walks into the kitchen, and puts water up for tea to have with the chocolate babka she baked the day before. She has been on her feet since morning, selling clothes at a Manhattan boutique.

"Would you like a cup of tea, Ben?" she asks in her still-thick Eastern European accent.

Ben abruptly rises from the sofa, walks over to his mother, and throws her onto the floor, saying, "Why do you keep baking my cake with poison?"

The next week, Mr. and Mrs. X bring Ben to Rosedale Hospital. When asked why they have brought him in for admission, they say, "He has not talked in six years." That's all. No mention of either the car or cake incident. When Ben is asked why he's there, all he says is, "Everything is fine."

It's the end of a hard summer, and I've just driven almost three hours south to get to work at Rosedale. My mother died a few months ago, and the ride down gives me a stretch of time to maybe think about it. This summer I've been writing a lot of poems and have been generally withdrawn.

I unlock the door to the ward and walk down the hall toward the nurses station. A new patient is standing motionless next to the water fountain. He gazes at the wall and doesn't seem to notice me as I pass. No matter how distracted I am, there's no way I could miss him. His looks arrest me. More than six feet tall, with a lean build, he has close-cropped black hair and piercing dark eyes, a long, aquiline nose, and full lips. He's wearing an immaculately tailored shirt tucked in to bleached blue jeans and plain white sneakers. As I walk by, I'm uncomfortably aware of how small I am compared with his large frame. A nurse on duty tells me Ben has just come on the ward and barely talks.

The next day, he's standing in the exact same place, staring at the same spot on the wall. I stop.

"Hi. My name is Karen Chase, and I write poems with people here. I'm wondering if you'd like to try it."

"Yes," he says, without moving his eyes from the wall. Surprised that he answered me, and surprised that he agreed, I set up a time to meet with him the following week.

Before this, I'd worked with a few people at Rose-dale who were silent or almost silent. It took enormous will and wish on both my part and the patient's part to make a go of it. Ben's first definitive yes and my suscep-tibility at that moment made for an auspicious start.

Since my mother's death in the spring, I had pulled back from the hospital work. Each week when I ar-rived there, the staff, out of concern and compassion, asked how I felt, how I was doing. Really, I had noth-ing to say, but I responded, "Things are going okay." What had been okay, in fact, was writing. It was my sanctuary.

Talking about her death was not what I wanted to do. In fact, talking about anything had little appeal. So when the staff told me that Ben said the words "yes," "no," "everything is fine," and rarely anything else, that sounded mighty good to me.

The next week, I'm due to meet with Ben for the first time. I wake up early in my cottage on a lake in rural Massachusetts. In the coming light of morning, I make my way out to the cold, dark car, turn the heat way up, leave the radio off, and begin the long drive south. No thoughts of Ben — in fact, no thoughts at all. The ride passes in a flash. There I am, pulling into the huge hospital parking lot. Where have I been all these hours? I have no idea. Fumbling through my oversize canvas bag for my keys as I meander through the lav-ish corridors, then up the stairs to the ward, I find my furry rabbit's foot on the key chain. I unlock the heavy ward door. Ben is watching the weather report on TV at the end of the hall. His eyes land right on me, and he gets up and walks in my direction. I motion toward the porch and say hi. He says nothing, and we both walk to the porch.

The "porch" is a long, narrow room with a bank of windows facing the enormous old maples outside. On the opposing wall, a large plate-glass window looks in to the nurses station. More accurately, the window looks out; whatever happens on the porch is visible to the staff, and they keep watch. Today I'm particularly aware and glad about this. It's windy, I notice as I walk in and sit down. The leaves look very huge and very green. I'm aware of the discrepancy between the outside lushness and the inside drabness.

Ben sits down, then I sit on a chair on the opposite side of a long, low oak table. Neither of us has uttered a sound so far, but it is strangely comfortable.

As if it were one vague, long word, I mumble, "Whatdoyouthinkofpoetry?"

As I ask the question, Ben averts his eyes, then focuses right on me. His look turns into the definition of eye contact. He says nothing.

"You like it?" I ask.

Long pause, tense again. Still, oddly comfortable.

"No."

Now Ben glares at me, as if the sound of my voice has insulted him. *He did agree to meet with me,* I remind myself, a bit confused.

"Want to write?" I say.

"Yes."

Here is a man who says little, but he seems to say what he means. I lean over and pull a small stone from my briefcase. Because he looked like a stone to me the week before, it occurred to me that we might use a stone as a takeoff for writing.

I call the stone the "third thing." When I first began to teach at Rosedale, there were numerous objects—you could call them ritual objects—that I brought in to stimulate writing. Put an apple, a shoe, a shell on a table, and each writer can focus on it in his or her written line.

When I put the stone on the table between us, Ben did not touch the stone but looked at it for a long while. I wrote, "I am a stone" on top of the page and handed him the pad and pencil. Neither of us said a word. Without a moment's hesitation, he wrote, "a stone is good" and passed the pad back to me. I added another line. And so began the rhythmic back and forth of our work together, a reliable pattern that lasted for two years.

I am a stone (K)
a stone is good (B)
it sits on a field (K)
it never worries (B)
it never dreams (K)
it always comes through (B)
in any weather (K)
everything is always fine with it (B)

even in blizzards (K)
everything is always okay with a stone (B)

By relating to the "third thing," the stone, rather than to each other or ourselves, I wanted to stress that our writing was going to be about the outside world, that we were not going to use words to directly express anything personal. As a psychiatric patient, he was continually urged to talk about his personal life. As a woman who had just lost her mother, I was often urged to talk about her death, with the assumption being that talking about my loss would help.

Writing poems with Ben was going to be different. I wanted to show this stonelike character that external images can correspond to internal states. Writing about a stone was a way to be personally accurate, a way to tell a subjective truth. In other words, I'm not really a stone, but I'm like a stone. When I wrote "I am a stone," I was telling Ben, You can make up things in a poem, and I was saying, You're not alone, fellow. I, too, could be stony.

Much like Ben's posture, the structure of his lines was rigid. Although my lines respond to his, the reverse is not true. You can read his lines and skip over mine. Had he ignored what I wrote? I had no idea.

Even if he was ignoring my lines, my experience of writing our poem was vastly different from my work with Ashley, another patient on the ward. After I wrote my line, she traced over it as if it were hers. When I wrote another, she erased it and replaced it with a different one. It took a long while before we alternated with our own lines. The notion of dialogue had been absent. For her, talking meant monologue, and she talked incessantly. Talking seemed to be her way to fill space, to erase other people.

But with Ben, I sensed connection from the start. Perhaps it was the genuineness of his words, few though they were, and his intent face. This, coupled with the space that silence provided, gave me a chance to imagine connection whether it was there or not.

In this first collaborative poem, "I Am a Stone," Ben started the lengthy process of teaching me how to talk or, in this case, write to him and how he chose or was able to use words or not.

In the week between my first and second meeting with Ben, I was back home in the Berkshires, spending the days writing poems related to my mother and her death. As Virginia Woolf indicated, "Writing dulls the sledgehammer blows of life," which is exactly what I was doing. Thoughts of Ben were far from my mind.

A few months earlier, on my first day back at work after my mother died, I had walked to the formal gardens on the spacious, luxurious hospital grounds, which was designated a historic landmark. For a while, I sat on a stone bench surrounded by tall yellow roses. It was early in the day, with moisture in the air and dew still on the grass. The smell of roses was overwhelming. I was wearing my mother's khaki safari jacket, which I had just taken from her closet. She, who had been one cold character, felt close—her jacket on my skin.

I sat on the bench and daydreamed of driving home, packing up my possessions, loading up my car, and returning to the hospital to live. I found a scrap of paper in the jacket pocket and scrawled notes for a poem.

Finally, I made my way back to the ward to meet with a patient named Joe. I brought a box of pastel crayons to our meeting. He chose a gray crayon and handed it to me. I scribbled a mass of gray on the page. He smelled the page, said it reminded him of me, then began to write. He smelled the page, wrote some more. At the end of our time, he asked whether he could keep the page, then walked from the room, smelling it. The sight was striking. The smell of the crayon page for Joe seemed similar to the sensation of my mother's jacket on my skin, each object a substitute for a person's presence. I think my mother's death helped me better understand how the patients felt, and I think this mental opening paved the way for my work with Ben.

As I drove south to meet Ben for the second time, my mind filled with thoughts and images of him, far from the blankness of the previous drive. Before I went to the ward to begin work, I stopped at the patient-run canteen for hot chocolate and a bagel. When I picked up the bagel, a funny mental-health worker with crumbly muffin in hand blurted out, "Can't deal with chewing today; I'll pass on a bagel."

I drank my hot chocolate, hoping to calm down, then went to the ward. When I unlocked the door, Ben was waiting right on the other side. Hi, I said, and together we wordlessly trooped to the porch as if we had been doing this for years. Our habits were forming.

I hadn't planned what we would write about, intending to take my cue from Ben. Sometimes I like to rely on my response at the moment to come up with a writing idea, much as a musician improvises when playing. I sense what is going on with the other person and with myself at the time and take into account what we wrote in our last meeting.

This time Ben and I sat down on metal folding chairs side by side but at a distance, with the oak table in front of us. His chiseled features were set in position; his face looked polished like a statue. We didn't face each other but rather looked at the page in front of us or out the window at a tree. I was nervous and trying not to be.

I handed Ben a typed copy of our poem from the previous week. He took it, read it to himself. As I watched his eyes race across the page, I remembered that a nurse had said he was a prize-winning runner in junior high school. His eyes moved from left to right, then back again—a vision of contained motion. It was as if his mind were sprinting but his body was fixed in position. Something about this sight struck a chord in me, but I had no idea what it was.

"Would you like a copy of the poem? I made one for you."

"No."

I got the hint. I didn't ask him if he would like to begin the next poem. It seemed clear the answer was no.

So I took the white, lined pad and pencil and focused completely on the page. No thoughts. Then, instinctively, quickly, I scribbled, "I live in Iceland." I used images of glaciers in my lines to cool my nervousness, to moderate my increasingly strong reaction to Ben.

After Ben had been in the hospital for a few months, an outside psychiatrist was consulted on his case, as was the custom. Every few months, a patient's situation was reviewed in front of the staff at a case conference. Prior to the conference, a written protocol was prepared by staff members from different departments, including myself, summarizing their work with the person. The day of the conference, the consulting psychiatrist interviews the patient in front of the staff, the patient returns to the ward, and then discussion begins. Usually the psychiatrist in charge is kind and respectful to the patient being interviewed. Still, it is a difficult, if not awful, position to be in for any person, particularly one who closely guards his or her privacy.

Ben walks into the conference room staring straight ahead. The consulting doctor extends his hand to Ben and introduces himself. They shake hands. The psychiatrist is a large, relaxed-looking fellow in a too-baggy brown suit. I'm relieved he's not the perfect-fitting blue-pinstriped type with an invasive look. Rather, he looks like a large, sweet mammal.

When he begins to talk to Ben, Ben fixes his eyes on him. He appears to take the doctor's questions to heart. He looks thoughtful, as if he is considering each question fully.

11

Yes, he says to some questions.

No, he says to others.

He utters no other words.

One of the summaries for the case conference reported that when Ben was asked by his peers why he didn't talk to them, he said, "I prefer not to." The staff member continued, "When they pursue this and ask why not, the patient does not answer." What had happened between the time he was kicked out of high school for talking too much and now?

Ben left the conference room, escorted back to the ward by a male nurse. What, I wondered, did he think of the procedure?

"In another time, Ben might have been considered a saint," the doctor began. "His sphinxlike look, his piercing black eyes, his statuesqueness, his few words, each offered as if it is monumental—his authentic manner reflects a purity of belief."

One day Ben paces back and forth in the hallway, as was his wont. He goes to the bathroom to scrub his hands, then goes back out to pace the hallway. Half an hour later, he returns to the bathroom to wash his hands again. He doesn't say anything to anyone as he alternates between hall-walking and hand-washing. The third time he returns to the bathroom, he opens the door and sees a fellow patient, a young man who lives in the room adjacent to Ben's, nearly dead and hanging from the ceiling. Ben washes his hands and leaves the bathroom. He proceeds to walk the hallways once again. He doesn't utter a word about what he has just witnessed. Later, when he's questioned about this, he says he didn't see it.

Ben denies seeing much that goes on in the ward. When he's asked about scaring a fellow patient at a volleyball game by smiling strangely, he claims it never happened. When he's asked about the fact that his father is drunk when he brings him back from outside passes, he says it's not true. In fact, Ben denies anything bad that happens. But compared with the near suicide he witnessed and denied, these examples are mild. His silence reached extremes.

By the time Ben had been in the hospital for nearly a year and a half, he was speaking, although sparsely. One day, a new patient on the ward, with no buildup or warning, simply walked over to a table, picked it up, and threw it into a barred window. Emergency buzzers blared. In a flash, six large male staff members materialized and carried the struggling new fellow to what is called the "quiet room."

The quiet room is a small, windowless room, fifteen feet by twelve, with padded walls and a padded floor. The door to the hallway has a small window so that staff can constantly monitor the person inside. Patients are put there to calm down when they're out of control. It's isolated and physically safe, both for the patient and other people on the ward.

The following day, Ben told his therapist about the

incident. He thought it was good, he said, that the man had been put in the quiet room because it kept him under control. Ben initiated the exchange about something obviously important to him, and as far as I know, it was the only time he did that.

Is the quiet room, symbolically, where Ben placed himself by not speaking? Perhaps his silence was a way of containing what he feared he'd say or do if he spoke. Had he learned from his family to stay quiet about devastating experiences?

Sometime during World War II, when they were young teenagers, Ben's Jewish parents had emigrated from Poland to the United States. They later moved their young family to Israel. The consulting psychiatrist for Ben's case conference after a year and a half of hospitalization thought their war experience may have played some part in Ben's silence. What follows is an excerpt from his notes describing his interview of Ben prior to the conference.

War had spread to all of Europe by 1940, at a time when Ben's father was 13. One glaring omission from this otherwise complete report is anything related to the parents' war experience. It is simply mentioned that they are holocaust survivors, but there is a total blank in the family history for those years.

In my interview with Ben yesterday, I asked him if his parents ever talked about this time in their lives. An otherwise desultory interview became very tense. He stared at me. He stared at the floor. His jaw muscles rippled. He said no, they never did. I said never. He said never. I asked how his parents met. He said he did not know. He thought it was in Europe. I pressed for details. He said he thought it had something to do with the war. There was a long pause.

Then Ben said, "Once, my father told me that all the effects of the war had worn off."

Ben was unable to remember exactly when that conversation was or any more about it. When I asked if he was curious about what his father meant or about that time, he again stared at me—paused a long time, and then said no.

Silence, or at least a hesitance to talk, is seen differently in different families and different cultures. In the tiny culture of Ben's family, perhaps silence was valued.

In some cultures, silence is expected in certain situations. Sometimes, "it is right to give up on words." A Western Apache from Arizona explained that when strangers meet, silence is traditional. As opposed to the Western Apaches, the Swampy Cree from Canada view silence as abnormal. In their oral tradition, children are given names based on stories about them, and the story/poems are passed along. The following poem ("Quiet Until the Thaw" from *The Wishing Bone Cycle: Narrative Poems from the Swampy Cree*, edited and translated by Howard Norman) explains why a girl was called Quiet Until the Thaw:

Her name tells of how
it was with her.

The truth is, she did not speak
in winter.
Everyone learned not to
ask her questions in winter
once this was known about her.

The first winter this happened
we looked in her mouth to see
if something was frozen. Her tongue
maybe, or something else in there.

But after the thaw she spoke again
and told us it was fine for her that way.

So each spring we
looked forward to that.

The tolerance and respect the people have for her silent ways shows in the second stanza. Their concern, coupled with their wish to discover the cause for her silence, shows in the third. Finally, they take her at her word and are relieved that each spring she speaks again.

When I read this poem aloud, one patient blurted out, "Here the doctors would say she has seasonal affective disorder!"

In the culture of our new millennium, silence has no place at all. To speak freely and in detail about one's intimate experiences is commonplace, even expected. But during the decade I worked at Rosedale, such easy, intimate talk was less common in the general culture. On the ward, however, such personal talk was encouraged and highly valued. Patients and staff discussed one another and the ward in community meetings. Patients met among themselves to discuss issues important to them. Patient treatment was discussed in peer groups. In nursing one-on-ones, patients talked with their assigned nurses about practical problems. In psychotherapy sessions, patients explored personal matters with their doctors. And social workers, families, and patients tackled family problems by talking.

Although there was strong emphasis on discussion, it came hard to many of the patients. Some spoke with ease but did not stand behind their words; their words lacked meaning. One bright patient spoke with unusual ease, but his voice seemed to originate at a distance from his body, like the puppet of a ventriloquist. Other patients like Ben spoke very little or not at all.

A unique aspect of my poetry meetings with the patients was the assumption that talk was beside the point. Writing poems was the point. All kinds of people, regardless of who they are or where they're from, often find they love writing poems. As Emerson said, "The man is only half himself, the other half is his expression." When you scratch the surface, the desire for expression is found in surprising places—it's nearly everywhere. Once a person chooses to write poems to express him or herself, I believe the poems belong to that person only, to do what he or she wants with them.

When I first began at Rosedale, I had to battle with certain staff members about what it meant to be a "poet-in-residence" in a mental hospital. One day I attended a staff meeting led by a renowned psychiatrist. When one patient was being discussed, she asked me to describe the subject matter of a poem the patient had just written. Then she suggested that the patient's psychotherapist use the material in the poem as a way to probe the patient's psyche. Although I was an unknown outsider at that point, I gritted my teeth and spoke up, explaining that in my work with the patients, they understand that their poems are their property. If they want to show them to anyone, that's fine. If they want to rip them up and throw them away, that's fine too. Of course, if a patient's poem implied physical danger to anyone, I would immediately alert staff. Otherwise, their poems would not be passed along to staff as a takeoff point for discussion about their lives. Because writing—or earlier in my life, painting—had always been my sanctuary, I held these notions near and dear.

Then I asked a therapist what she would think if I took the substance of a patient's dream they had just discussed and used it for the starting point for writing a poem with the patient.

I believe that the poet's job on the ward is particular. Therapists, of course, have their own particular and crucial job with patients. And these two approaches should not be blurred because the jobs are different and occasionally in conflict.

For me, these were tense times. I was making my way in a foreign setting with stubborn beliefs. Rather than dilute those beliefs, I would have preferred to go elsewhere to do the work. Yet I was aware that few people knew me and because of that had good reason to question my judgment. In fact, that renowned psychiatrist asked me not to work on her ward after that meeting. I did not belong there. Patient treatment on that ward was highly invasive, and while that approach helped some people, it was the wrong place for me to do this particular work.

The introduction of a poet into the Rosedale ranks had been a paradox. In the 1960s, psychiatric patients were commonly offered art, music, dance, and drama therapies, reflecting the expansiveness and experimentation of that time. But with the widespread use of effective medications, vocational rehabilitation and social-skills improvement were emphasized. Returning patients to the community as quickly as possible became the primary goal. By welcoming a poet as a worker, the hospital went back to an earlier tradition but in a new way. The clinicians wondered if poetry writing would increase communication skills, which might aid patients in their daily lives. Instead of being an arts therapist integrated into the hospital system, I was there as a poet to offer an outsider's view. Some staff members were curious to see how writing poetry would affect the patients. Some romanticized the idea of having a poet-in-residence on the ward. Some were simply skeptical.

Soon after I left that first ward, I was introduced to Ann, another well-known psychiatrist who was the head of a different ward. We spent a long time exchanging ideas and mulling over our beliefs. At the end of the meeting, she announced, "You have my blessing." She was an inspired and inspiring teacher about why human beings act the way they do. Her wide-ranging, generous view of people and her respect for each person made for a unique, productive atmosphere for both patients and staff.

When I first walked onto Ann's ward for people with severe mental illness in 1980, I entered an unusual setting. Patients could expect to remain there for one to three years; on other wards they returned to the community in a month or two. Psychotherapy was stressed, although patients also received medication. With the staff, these patients, mostly in their mid- to late twenties, actively participated in their own and one another's treatment in order to foster a sense of self-determination and community.

At that point, a psychiatrist named Dennis, who was in charge of a large part of the hospital, became my supervisor. Little did I know then how complex the supervisory relationship with him would become.

Language, I believe, comes about in reaction to contact and with a sense of urgency, regardless of any particular setting or family or culture. For many months, Ben and I said few words out loud to each other. One day, while reading him our poem during an early meeting, he fixed his eyes on my mouth. Perhaps he had done this before, but this time I was aware of it. I continued to read, sensing Ben was registering me in a new way, that is, sexually. I felt self-conscious.

"That's a good one," Ben blurted out when I finished reading the poem. His words startled me.

That evening, I played with the infant son of a friend. Looking at his face, I made funny noises. "Eeeeeeeee. Ooooooooo. Mummummuuummumm." The baby fixed his eyes on my mouth. Then, he made his own sounds. "Ooooooooooo. Ehhhhhhhhh." The interplay between us, the intentness of his gaze, and then the sounds we each formed made me think about my meeting with Ben earlier that day. What I took as sexuality might not have been at all what Ben felt. In fact, it was what I felt. Often I realized that I couldn't know what was going on inside him.

Working with Ben elicited primitive emotions—violence, sex, murder—at night while I dreamed. But for the most part, I was neither scared of Ben nor aware of a sexual undercurrent. In the daytime, during our meetings, I was calm, collected, and acutely focused on our work.

One night I dreamed I was at a Rosedale Christmas party in a big house. Wherever Dennis went, I went too. I sat on his lap, our bodies draped around each other. Ben strode into the house, walked straight up to me, cornered me in a kitchen, and said, "You cunt." I bolted outside onto a spacious wraparound porch.

My sons were in the house, and Ben was going to kill them. I couldn't figure out how to warn them without riling him up so that he would end up killing me, them, and other people. I looked around, saw some nurses, and told them to get an ambulance to take Ben away.

The ambulance pulled up. Uniformed men went in the house and came out leading Ben, who was wrapped in restrictive white hot packs, like what I had been wrapped in when I was a girl with polio.

I took care to reveal my flashes of fear and my hospital-related dreams to Dennis. Having an unusually sensitive supervisor made it possible for me to proceed with a mix of extreme consciousness about certain aspects of the work—language, poetry, silence—and relative unconsciousness about others. Someone solid was overseeing the murky underside of the work, freeing me to spontaneously write poems with Ben. Because poems often spring to life from the unconscious, this ingredient was critical. If I had had to always keep in mind the depth and intensity of what was happening between Ben and me, I wonder now if I could have done the work and if it would have been as fruitful.

Although Ben and I barely spoke when we began, my attention almost never wavered. I registered almost every move Ben made in his writing and actions. My attention came from my wish to understand and make contact with this seemingly unreachable but intriguing person. Although Ben was the patient and I was the staff member, we were two human beings in the same place at the same time, embarked on this unusual journey.

Because of their genuineness, I call what Ben and I wrote *poems*. But, for the most part they would not be considered "good" poems. Only a few attended to sound and rhythm. There was very little play with words, very few leaps in meaning. Gradually he became interested in the subject of poetry. After the first year, when we began to speak a bit, Ben and I mentioned elements of poetry like the sound of words, their rhythm. He slowly began to show glimmerings of understanding about how to use language to express his personal vision of the world.

He introduced talk after about three months of work together. Gradually, there was a bit more talk, and his writing became more expressive. Meanwhile, I maintained steady conditions. We met in the same place at the same time, no surprises. The steadiness provided a predictable atmosphere for growing expression and contact between us, as well as safety and comfort for two people with an unpredictable, powerful task.

When Ben finally began to speak, his words were about our poems, and that was how we made verbal contact. Once I wrote the line, "Sometimes it's unseasonably warm." When I read the poem aloud to Ben, as was our habit, I expected silence.

Instead, he piped up, "Is there any reason *particularly* that you chose *warm*?"

Flabbergasted, I replied, "I don't know. . . . Let me think for a second. I guess it was because yesterday was unseasonably warm. . . . And also because of what we wrote last week. I suppose it's a combination of the outside world [I pointed out the window] and the inside world."

While at Rosedale, I taught hundreds of patients, both individually and in workshops, and read thousands of their poems. Provocative, compelling questions arose. How does language and expressiveness develop or redevelop in severely ill people when they write poems? Does collaborative poetry writing influence this verbal expansion? Why do people who otherwise shun contact with others often make contact when writing poems? Patients who did not speak or spoke very little sometimes allowed themselves to write poems. Over time, some began to speak.

After four months into our work, one winter day I handed Ben a fragment of worn blue crockery to use for our writing. "I was turning the soil for my garden early last spring," I said, "and I found this piece of a broken plate in the dirt, which I liked. I thought you might be wondering what it was."

Revealing this bit of personal information was a leap, but by then Ben had exhibited signs of curiosity, so I chose to say what I did. It was the first time I told him something personal and the first time he imaginatively used language.

The crockery looks very old (B)
from a bowl in someone's kitchen (K)
it has a very smooth texture (B)
smooth close up, smoothness
from a distance (K)

it appears to be delicate (B)

it's something to keep
I'll call it a "keeper" (K)
it's a hot weather stone (B)

As he stared at the crockery, as I picked it up and put it down, noticing its smoothness, he wrote, "it has a very smooth texture." When I wrote, "smooth close up, smoothness from a distance," I mentioned us both as observers, feeling intertwined with him at that moment. As I was physically handling the shard, he was describing it. Ben fixed his eyes on me, then away.

So, when he wrote, "it appears to be delicate," I sensed he was saying I seemed delicate. His use of the word *appears* was subtle and exacting, suggesting delicacy as well.

Keeping pace with him, I wrote, "it's something to keep, I'll call it a keeper," implying that the crockery and furthermore his reaction mattered to me. Then Ben added, "it's a hot weather stone," transforming the crockery into a stone with imaginative qualities. Things had gotten personal, and for the first time he used his imagination by returning to our first image, a stone. The circuit of language and interplay between us was complete that day.

I was becoming more aware of my own intimate reaction to Ben the week we wrote our crockery poem. I had been listening to Billie Holiday records and was reading an essay ("Billie Holiday and Lester Young on 'Me, Myself, and I'") by the poet William Matthews about Holiday and the saxophonist Lester Young. He wrote:

> When they worked together, they were continually finishing each other's musical sentences. . . . His solos are studded with oddly accurate silences, often at the beginning of a phrase. It's as if the listener has come into a sentence halfway through. By the end it will be complete and full of feeling. For the length of time it takes Holiday to sing the eight lines of threadbare lyrics again and Young to play along, all those usual silences in his solos are filled by Holiday singing. At times, she's singing and he's playing, both, like intertwined vines.

Listening over and over to the interplay of Holiday and Young on the cut "Fine and Mellow" nearly took my breath away, made me muse about the way Ben and I sometimes wrote together.

Change in Ben's surroundings worried him, so as much as possible we worked in the same place at the same time each week, although we changed locations several times in two years. In our first poem, "I Am a Stone," Ben wrote, "[a stone] never worries," "it always comes through," "everything is always fine with it," and "always okay with it." He used "always" and "never" twenty times in our first seven poems, showing how much he liked constancy.

Once, after only a few meetings, we had to meet off the ward in a different room. I became strangely jarred as we sat in unfamiliar chairs and without our usual table between us. I realized then how much the unusual silence in which we worked made me nervous and that I too counted on predictability. When I asked Ben if he liked meeting there, he emphatically said no.

What was this about? The silence of our meetings was unfamiliar elsewhere. Although Ben was steadfast in his speechlessness, when he was with other people he heard them speak to one another or they tried to get him to speak. He could hear the sound of voices, even if they were not his own. And I live in a world full of people talking, including myself. So, in general, our silence made for an intense and strange atmosphere rather than a noiseless, calm one. Each week, we sat in the same chairs, looked out the same window at the same tree. That sameness was like a tradition that helped lessen the tension between us. This is how it went.

I unlock the ward door and walk into the corridor. Ben is standing near the door, ready to meet. We walk to the porch and sit down. By then I have said hi, and sometimes so has he.

As we take our seats facing the oak table, I pull out the typed copies of the poems we have written the week before. I hand them to Ben. He reads them.

"Would you like to keep a copy of the poems?" I ask.

"No," he says.

His not wanting to keep poems often reminded me how much distance he required from anything that might evoke a strong reaction.

"Would you like to write today?"

"Yes," he answers.

To get things going, I often take some object from my bag as a writing stimulus or put on a music tape. I put the white, lined pad and pencil on the table.

"Do you want to start today or would like me to start?"

"You."

I pick the pad up and write a line, then hand it to Ben. He writes a line, then hands it to me. Rarely a word is uttered during the writing. I often notice that he reads all the lines from the top before he adds his. There is a calming rhythm to the back-and-forth, back-and-forth. Contact and distance are both in the air.

Our meetings last exactly thirty minutes. Precisely after fifteen minutes, Ben adds a line to the poem that clearly ends it. He always signals that he wants to write the last line.

"Do you want me to read it aloud?" I ask.

"Yes."

Slowly, I read our poem with no comment. His face lights up as he listens. As I continue to read, his muscles relax and sometimes his eyes warm up and sparkle.

"Do you like the poem?" I ask.

"Yes."

"Do you want it typed?"

"Yes."

In the dependable context of our work, Ben slowly began to make personal and linguistic moves. He initiated changes in our habits. After several months, sometimes he wrote the first line and sometimes I wrote the final one.

One day, I set a small piece of driftwood on the table to use for writing. He looked at it for a long while. Touching the object was rare. I chose not to say anything yet. Finally, as if he had decided to take a weighty act, he picked it up in his hands, examined it, and put it down.

"Would you like to start today or do you want me to start?" I asked.

"Either one," he said. Within a split second, he added, "I choose water," picked up the pad and pencil, and wrote, "water is really cold."

From that day forward, there was flexibility about who would begin. On the other hand, he ignored my rare efforts to introduce anything new into the repetitive structure of our work. There was no doubt about it—Ben was in charge of change.

During our first year, we sometimes wrote like each

other, switching styles. Although we alternated lines, I might feel peculiarly blank and the only line I could think of would sound oddly like Ben's. Perhaps this was a way for us to discover how each other felt. Once I wrote, "everything ices up," then feeling frozen and blank, I mumbled "I can't think of anything." In turn, he too wrote lines that sounded like mine. I wrote, "Flying with the geese," to which he added, "across the tremendous distance of sky" and then continued, "flowers stretch across the field." Was he trying his hand at being expansive?

Our habit of writing alternate lines continued the entire time we met. Within that structure, Ben's own voice became more distinct. Our lines responded more to each other's and became more lively. Exactly a year after we began meeting, we wrote a poem in which Ben, dramatically, took my position.

For the few days prior to that meeting, I had been having a rough stretch. I had been up much of the night before, awakened by dreams about my mother's illness and death a year and a half earlier. The drive from my house down to the hospital seemed to take forever. It took every bit of concentration to stay awake and focus on the road. I drank coffee before I got in the car and stopped for more on the way. I kept being tempted to close my eyes as I was driving. I considered turning around, going home, and calling in sick. Passing farms, I saw a corn silo, and I remembered how the amount of corn had diminished each week when my mother was dying. At that point, I had been driving to

New York City every few days to see her. My exhaustion overtook me, so I pulled over, took a quick nap, and then set out again toward the hospital.

Miraculously not late, I finally arrived on the ward. There was Ben, pacing up and down the hall, staring at the ceiling as he paced. My mind was elsewhere. I wanted to go home—a first during our work together. As usual, we walked to the porch and sat down at the table.

"Why don't you pick a topic and begin?" Ben pipes up as I am about to begin our usual exchange.

Stunned by his sentence, stunned by the authority with which he says it, I wonder if he is as tuned in to me as I am to him. He is acting like the teacher. Do I look vulnerable? Do I seem out of reach this time? I look out the window at the sky and then write, "Layers of pink stripe the sky." Then I add, "Black birds crash through the sky / speeding south."

In response to my obviously distraught lines and my facial expression, Ben ends the poem with "The colors of the sky together / combine to form a colorful / array of light." His words—"together," "combine," "form," "array"—are tender.

Quietly, I read the poem aloud, and our meeting time ends. Neither of us says a word or moves for what must have been about a minute. Then he gets up and leaves. I feel paralyzed for a few minutes. Later, in supervision, as I describe to Dennis what happened, I wonder how Ben, the man who half an hour earlier seemed to live in such a distant realm, pacing and pacing, was able to come forward in such a human, humane way.

Col means together, *labor* means work. *Collaboration* is working together. It is an unusual way to write a poem and an unusual way to communicate. In this unusual structure of sitting down each week together, barely speaking, and then alternating lines of poems, many things happened. Ben could express the irrational, hard as that was for him. Only rarely did he allow himself the flexibility to veer from the concrete or the linear. One time, he wrote, "the wind is bruising the tree branch." As usual, I read the poem aloud, but when I said "bruising," he interrupted me to say he had misspelled the word, that he had intended to write "brushing." Yet he was a nearly perfect speller.

Then I noticed the stone on the shelf that we sometimes used for writing and thought how it was like a weapon. My fear of Ben's past violence surfaced for a moment. Usually, I simply did not think of his violent history. We met in safe places, and the staff thought he was trustworthy. But every once in a while, I was aware that his silence camouflaged extraordinarily strong emotions and I didn't know what they were.

At the same time that he was registering our distinctiveness, he also took pleasure in our link. One day he listened as I read aloud the poem we had just written. "I like it," said Ben, and then after a long pause, "the lines go into one another like they are continuous."

I think it was his way of saying our lines were paying attention to each other, that *we* were paying attention to each other. We had come far from our first poem, in which Ben's lines paid no heed to mine, where there was no apparent link, and all he said out loud was yes or no. Now our lines were sometimes in tune with each other's and other times not. In either case, he was sometimes brought to speech by this.

One time it became clear that our lines did not follow each other's. I wrote, "it was a green sea." He added, "the water being a tremendous blue color." Caught off guard, I questioned him.

"I don't get it. Could you tell me if the water is blue or green?"

He grabbed the page back, reread it, and became flustered.

"I didn't read your line before I wrote mine," he said. He boldly crossed his line out, getting rid of the colors, and quickly scrawled, "the water was rolling along all day." His face flushed red.

The Alarmingness of Red
Color and Expression

Ben was in the shower when I got to the ward. By now, after a year's work, this was not uncommon. He was almost always either ready at the door or off in the shower when I arrived, either waiting for contact or seemingly avoiding it.

But this day, he was unusually late. Finally, I went to his room to see if he was there, a bold move. I had never looked inside his door before. His room had the usual bed, dresser, and desk. It was a stark sight. The room looked like a white shell before someone moved in. Blanket and sheets were pulled tight across the bed. The words *hospital corners* never had such an odd ring when I saw how perfectly executed they were. No object on the dresser top, no object on the desk. *What did Ben use the desk for*, I wondered. Nothing on the walls. Because every room on the ward had framed posters decorating the walls, he must have removed them. Then I remembered learning that Ben threw out any object he was given—books, slippers, a comb. The barrenness of the room was like Ben's language when we first met: no trace revealed.

In his room, one large window looked out on the grand hospital lawn. Seeing the open green expanse and thinking of Ben made me recall something M. F. K. Fisher wrote: "Probably one of the most private things in the world is an egg until it is broken."

Ben kept his clothes tidy in his closet and refused to do his laundry on the ward. His mother insisted on washing his clothes at home.

After his shower, Ben, dressed immaculately in his jeans and blue shirt, walked down the hall. His brand-new white sneakers had a thin bright strip of red near the soles. How cheered I was to see that bit of red after viewing his lifeless room.

We walked to the porch saying nothing, which was a bit awkward. His long stretch in the shower, my boldly looking in his room, and then his fresh appearance all made me think, *This is like a first date.* Early in our time together, I would not have allowed myself such an unbuttoned thought, but at this point my work with Ben felt solid.

We sat down and he wanted me to begin. All along, our poems had mentioned colors, but this poem, which I introduced, was the first that concentrated on color. The poem begins:

Imagining colors (K)
blue is very dark (B)

Ben wrote about color over and over again; only weather appeared more often. Mention *red*, mention *yellow*, mention the word *green*, and Ben's language took on expressiveness. I was not surprised to learn that he had liked art as a grammar-school boy. And it was not surprising that his parents reported Ben liked his art teacher. Perhaps the chance for artistic expression was a reason he initially agreed to write poems.

Exploring Ben's changing use of color shows how his language became more and more moving. As I looked at how Ben used color, I could not help but think how much I love color.

My mother had been an abstract painter; her canvases were masses of vibrant color. She taught me the color wheel the way most children are taught the alphabet.

When I was four, she took me on long train rides to New York City to a painting class in the basement of the Metropolitan Museum of Art. When the train crossed the Harlem River Bridge, I would look down at the moving water and know we were getting closer to painting class; my excitement would rise to a new pitch.

But it was Ben, in fact, who started introducing color into our poems, and he ended up mentioning it more than twice as often as I did. Although I'll never know whether he would have mentioned color so often on his own, whether he sensed my attraction to it, or whether my interest awakened something alive in him already.

Ben continued to teach me how to talk to him in "Imagining Colors"—what the right distance was, what happened when I moved too quickly, too surprisingly, or too intensely. He also showed what happened when I understood him. I had to be like a drummer, on top of the beat or right on it, to keep the momentum going and the interest growing.

Imagining colors (K)
blue is very dark (B)
when no light hits it (K)

Yellow is very nice (B)
on a cab, on a canvas (K)

Red is Alarming (B)
Red (K)

These colors are always
around, they brighten up
everything and liven everything up (B)

Up with color (K)

Red goes very fast
it always goes fast
and is very lively (B)

Zooming red (K)

Things Always come alive
When Red is there (B)

You can live in the color red (K)

Colors can sometimes Be Very Dark (B)

You wade through them
like through a swamp (K)

They are always pleasant (B)
they're okay (K)

They sometimes fill the
Air with a bright glow (B)
blueness (K)

They always shine on
alarming everything (B)

A few weeks earlier, I had used *yellow* in our poem. Then Ben dashed off "things strike out." Something— was it the color?—had evoked a strong swift reaction with a tinge of violence from him.

"The poem was quick. It was very yellow," he said when we were done.

So when he wrote "Yellow is very nice" in "Imagining Colors," I wondered whether he was scared of color

floating free in the imagination. I thought he used *nice*
to offset his nervousness. At least it offset mine.

I wanted to make color seem safer, so I attached
yellow to concrete objects—a cab, a canvas. But Ben
was not eased. When he wrote, "Red is Alarming" to
emphasize his point, he used capital letters for the
first time. I was excited by his display, by the capital *R*
and capital *A*. Careful though to keep a distance that
would not dampen his movement, I contained myself,
repeated *red*, trying to keep steady and reserved so he
would go further. Then Ben added:

> These colors are always
> around, they brighten up
> everything and liven everything up

Now Ben's language became lively and playful, with
the positioning of "up everything" and "everything up"
and the internal off-rhyme of "brighten" and "liven." In
the past, he used "always" and "everything" to deaden
impact. Now, with the same words, he's being lively
and playful! Here, the very thought of color produced
liveliness. The mood on the porch felt glittery.

One day during this time, midway in our work, I
began to register, then to crystallize, one huge aspect
of my work with Ben. I was home in the Berkshires,
taking a walk with my husband, Paul. We took this
route often, going around curves so you could not see
what was ahead or behind. Then a sweep of lake and
mountain came into view. A tangle of weeds grew

alongside the dirt road—bloodroot, overgrown honeysuckle, doll's eyes. It was early morning, the air chilly and moist, and we were chatting, moseying.

I walked over to the side of the road, careful of the lush poison ivy, to get a better look at some low-growing thing. In the brush was a cat. Its back was humped high into a steep arch; its eyes looked like bright blue marbles. It looked frozen. I was scared. We tried to get it to move, to blink. Then we walked on. After a few moments, we went back to the cat, hoping, I suppose, it would be gone. But the cat was still there, its fur straight on end as if it had been electrocuted. It was not breathing. The cat was dead.

We couldn't figure out what had happened. Had rigor mortis set in? That night, I could not get rid of the image of the frozen cat. Then my mind wandered over to Ben. He had seemed frozen for so many months after we met. Thoughts of my paralysis as a little girl with polio came to mind. I began to put some things together. I thought Ben's mental constriction was analogous to the physical constriction I felt as a child, unable to walk or move for a long time. Seeing the frozen cat was startling and forced these thoughts up to the surface.

Here's a psychiatrist's description of Ben's frozen look: "There was very little eye contact. His gaze would remain fixed to one side; however, it would furtively shift to me at times as though he had some curiosity about this other person in the room. The patient's strong appearance and silent presentation evoked reactions among the staff. Some staff saw him as 'a statue who communicated strength but said nothing.'"

Many people would be put off by such a character as Ben, his stance strange and even frightening. My time spent in a full-length plaster body cast—which people told me later was strange and frightening—and my paralyzed body made Ben's posture and bearing in some way familiar.

Ben was standing in the hallway motionless, his face expressionless, when I opened the locked ward door the week after "Imagining Colors." He looked the way he did when we first met. I was taken aback, because I had gotten used to a sense of nonverbal but reliable contact with him.

On days like this, our habits were particularly comforting and useful. We both knew what to do: walk to the porch, sit down. I hand him our poems from last week. He reads them and says nothing. Then, the usual exchange.

"Do you want copies?"

"No."

The pad and pencil sat on the low oak table.

"Do you want to begin?" I asked, fumbling in my bag for an old postcard to get us going.

"No. You begin. And write something out of the blue."

Out of the blue! He was asking me to use my imagi-

nation. I paused, collected myself, and thought a mo-
ment about how to proceed. Because of the jarring
shifts the week before, I set our next poem in a con-
tained place, as opposed to the boundless imagination.
If this poem was going to take a daring turn, let it be
Ben's choice.

"In a room," I wrote.

Ben took the pad and pencil, and as he did, his taut
posture relaxed, as if he were on familiar territory. He
added, "colors are everywhere."

In a room (K)

colors are everywhere (B)
on the four walls (K)

the room is well decorated (B)
proper (K)

It is alarming being in the
room because it is so colorful
It has Much Gray (B)

Each thing in the room
seems different (B)
we reach for silence (K)

It is a very good place (B)
to be, to ruminate (K)

It is Very Alive (B)
within that space (K)

And it looks Very good (B)
in its formality (K)

It is very well designed (B)
its color, its shape (K)

the different colors there
are very well chosen (B)

the size of the room
in careful proportion (K)

And so is everything in it (B)
cautious in color, shape, and
silence (K)

The room is Very exciting (B)
within those steady walls (K)

Was last week's "Imagining Colors" still on Ben's mind? His first line brought in color. Trying to tame the alarmingness of last week's poem, I contained the setting with "four walls." He echoed with "the room is well decorated," and I echoed with "proper."

Then Ben turned back to last week's color scare, adding "It is alarming being in the room / because it is so colorful." He sat up straight as if he were about to hand me the pad. Instead, he held onto it, looked down at it, and shuffled his feet. Wanting to seem casual, I looked out the window, then glanced over to him. He wrote, then gave me the pad and pencil. With a heavy hand, he had added, "It has Much Gray."

I was not thinking I had seen Ben's glaringly neutral room the week before. But as I read the poem later, I remembered. Surely when Ben wrote, "colors are everywhere," this was not his physical room. When he wrote how alarming it was to be in a room with so much color, he meant it. All his pausing and shuffling before he added "Much Gray" to the room made sense because, for Ben, bright color caused fear and neutral gray offered comfort. When we were done, as usual, I read the poem aloud.

"I like the writing of it," Ben said. "We've developed the writing to be very well. It's appealing to me, I don't know why."

A few hours later, Ben's therapist reported to me a comment Ben had made the day before. "How's poetry going?" he was asked.

"I've been having poetry for a long time and we've written a lot of poems. Now I think we're going to do something good."

Our world was contained—two people saying nothing or nearly nothing, intent on writing poems, handing a pad and pencil back and forth. There was a sense that we met in a vacuum, but another component to the work was my supervision.

When I first arrived at Rosedale, I was assigned a competent and helpful supervisor. He oversaw my work to ensure I was responsible and cautious. Because of my inexperience as a worker with psychiatric patients, this was essential and a relief. But eventually I wanted more. I wanted to collaborate with someone who was excited by the ideas that formed the work, who would add his or her own unique slant. I had heard about a particular psychiatrist, Dennis, with similar interests. So I sent him a note with a few patients' poems and a few thoughts. He responded with some of his own thoughts and ideas. His letter—open, funny, a little true, and a lot curious—helped start our supervisory collaboration.

Each week after I saw Ben, I would unlock the ward door, go to my office, and make copious notes of everything that had transpired in my meeting with Ben—every impression that had come my way, every single word spoken. Then I would rush down the stairs, down the long, carpeted corridors to Dennis's office. In minute detail, I would tell him what had just transpired between Ben and me. Then we would discuss the notes I had written the week before, after I had had the chance to mull them over. He always had fresh flowers in his office. He always had good coffee and milk waiting, and I needed it.

In much the same way Ben and I had our habits, Dennis and I had our own. I'd begin by reading him the two poems Ben and I had just written, without comment. Then we'd talk about anything that had happened in the meeting, anything either Ben or I had said. There was a flush about it all, energy glinting off the situation, going off and out for all three of us in different directions.

When people work well together in any realm — teacher and student, teammates, lawyer and client — they say the chemistry works. Whether it is intellectual, sexual, or psychological, chemistry is attraction. Attraction lends tension and impetus to the work. Certainly in the work Ben and I did, and the work Dennis and I did, there were myriad attractions.

There was a subtle playfulness between Ben and me the day we wrote the next poem, "Ordinary Indications." I wrote a line and handed the pad to Ben. As usual, he reread our work before he added his line. Normally when he did this, he kept the pad lower than his face, in a regular relaxed reading position. But this day he held the pad higher, so that his eyes were hidden by the pad. It looked effortful. This gave me a chance to watch him closely, uninhibited. He lowered the pad slowly, giving me time to avert my eyes. We had been working together for a year and a half, and this small shift made me realize the degree of sexual tension and play between us.

In the poem, our collaboration grew. While we each expressed what we wanted, which was sometimes at odds, we also paid close attention to what the other had written.

Ordinary indications —
coffee cups, curtains (K)

What a setting had been (B)
the kind of room to settle in (K)

It was calm and peaceful
yet loud (B), a bunch of daisies
in a vase (K)

Everything was going very fast (B)
a strong wind blew the curtains (K)

It was evening time and dark
there was much commotion and noise (B)
time to turn on the lamps (K)

There was a high mood of
orange in the room (B)

Set in the distant past, the poem's room is confusing, changeable, exciting, and troublesome. A slow, homespun atmosphere begins the poem, then turns fast and agitated. This contrasts to "In a Room," which was written in the present tense and in the end was a haven.

The framework for Ben's experience was growing. What was in his distant memory, I wondered, when he wrote, "what a setting had been." The past perfect tense usually refers to the earlier of two events, as if to say, "What a setting had been" for example, "before the storm came." The setting is placed not just in memory, but in buffered memory.

Ben's "it was calm . . . yet loud" changed the mood from quiet to tumultuous. So I focused on another detail of the room, flowers, and placed them in a vase, a symbol of containment.

At this moment, our writing picked up speed. One of us wrote a line, handed the pad to the other, who added a line and then handed it back. The rhythm quickened. When Ben further altered the mood, I followed his lead. Ben elaborated, expanded, "It was evening time and dark / there was much commotion and noise." His "commotion" seemed sexual. Without thought, I automatically scrawled, "time to turn on the lamps," as if I had actually turned the light on. To finish the poem, Ben kept the intensity with "a high mood" but brought in orange, the color of lamplight.

During this period, I had been painting and browsing through the *Complete Letters of Vincent Van Gogh* when I came upon a paragraph that made me think of Ben. In it, both color and words almost transcend what they stand for.

> Here's the description of a canvas in front of me at this moment. . . . This edge of the park is planted with large pine-trees, the trunks and branches being of red ocher, the foliage green darkened by a tinge of black. . . . You will realize that this combination of red ocher, green saddened by grey, and the use of heavy black outlines produces something of the sensation of anguish.

49

One day, I brought a box of colored pastels and sheets of blank white paper to fool around with before starting our poem. I asked Ben to pick a color he liked, and he chose blue. I scribbled a mass of blue on a blank white page and handed it to him.

"I'll have another," he said. He took the yellow from the box and handed it to me. He watched intently as I scribbled yellow on the page.

"I'll have another," he said and handed me the red.

Scribbling, I laughed and then said, "This is the best thing."

He looked at me as if he were almost charmed. He seemed fascinated watching me scribble. Suddenly, a new activity had been added to our repertoire.

My plan had been to use one of the colored pages as a takeoff for writing. But Ben was so intrigued with my scrawling colors that I discarded that idea.

"I'll have some scribbles," he said. He pondered the box of pastels for what seemed like a long time, then chose white.

He scribbled a mass of white on a white page. Then gray on another, then black on a third.

His scribbling movements exactly mimicked mine. It was remarkable how closely he had observed my physical motion.

"Do you want to see them?" he asked.

He wanted me to see his production.

"Yes!" I said, pleased.

"They're good. They're a good choice of colors. But I really wanted purple. But there wasn't any," he added in a monotone.

Red, yellow, blue—Ben chose the three primary colors, the colors that all others are made from, for me to use. Maybe he looked to me for something primary. Ben seemed to be saying important things through the metaphor of color.

Black, gray, white—for his own scribbles, he chose colorlessness. This was like his language, his room. But then Ben came forward and expressed a wish. He wanted purple, the distinguishing color of royalty and of mourning. At that moment, I took his comment to mean that he wished for something new.

Partly in response to his growing expressiveness, my reaction to him had changed. For more than a year, when we wrote our poems I rarely wondered about the facts of his life. I knew a few things but made no effort to learn others. Our time together was time to write—period. Our poems were the reality of the moment. For example, we once wrote about a boat trip in the middle of the ocean with a brilliant blue sky above, and I remember thinking afterward, *I've just been on a boat.* How vivid our time was in the compressed context of our writing. After our meetings, I would think about our poem and what had happened in the writing and go over it with Dennis. But apart from that, I would rarely think about Ben.

But now, although my time with Ben continued to focus on our writing, afterward I wondered more and more about him.

Towns filled with memories (K)
These memories lasted long (B)
their form changed (K)

There was
a lot of water nearby (B)
as if rivers could wash away
sounds (K)

It was easy to remember
them, the towns being so big
The sky would often be red (B)
unforgettable (K)

Memories usually changed but
these didn't seem to (B)
towns, sky, water hung on (K)

They were as good in modern
days as they were in the past (B)

Swift River, Red Sky, Bigness of Town (K)

Ben's lines made me wonder if he was remembering his boyhood in Israel. Had he been impressed by colorful skies? What made him write that memories "were as good in modern days as they were in the past?" Maybe he meant that particular memories or images—big towns or red skies—always had served him, had made a sanctuary in his mind.

Tel Aviv, of course, is on the Mediterranean Sea. Or did he live near the Dead Sea? And what about rivers—the Jordan River runs through the land, but I'm the one who introduced rivers, not Ben.

That day, a year and a half after we met, I was beset with curiosity about exactly where Ben had lived. I realized that although I was getting to know him very well in some ways, it was only through the writing. I knew very little about his life, so when he wrote about memories, I was provoked to wonder more about him.

When Dennis and I had our supervision meeting, we both wondered why I suddenly had become so curious about facts when the facts of Ben's life previously had been of little interest to me.

By now, Dennis had been supervising me for a long stretch. We discovered that our birthdays were both that week, so we decided to go out to celebrate. He lived on the hospital grounds and knew the neighborhood, knew a good place about ten minutes from the hospital where he liked to go. It was a dark bar with great hamburgers and beer, dartboards, and a pool table.

Sitting there in a maroon Naugahyde booth, trying to talk over the loud music, I told him that until I was five I lived in a town near the hospital but had never been back. In all the years of working nearby, it hadn't occurred to me how close it was. I told him we had lived on California Road, and he said: "It's right down

53

here! Just by the lake. Let's go there." After our meal, we took off in his car.

"California Road! Ahhh! There it is!"

And we drove around in the dark from one road to the next, and a town filled with memories came alive.

When I had first come to work at the hospital, a psychiatrist made a joke in a staff meeting: "I don't know if the patients are getting better, but we all sure are!" I laughed because I liked her irreverence, but I didn't actually grasp what she meant. That night, driving California Road with Dennis, I understood how fine it felt to have disparate parts of one's life woven together.

Ben's poems became more and more touching, but he never spoke or wrote directly about his life. Because his uttered speech remained sparse throughout his hospital stay, there remained a question about his diagnosis. In order to demonstrate a formal thought disorder such as schizophrenia, he would have had to be more open about what he thought. Many clinicians believed he was "significantly depressed." I wondered long after he left the hospital whether he ever would have wanted to speak of his life directly if he had written poems long enough, but I had no particular reason to think so. Because I worked with him as a poet, I kept encouraging expressiveness through metaphor, and in this way he grew.

One day, there was an emergency meeting that had to take place on the porch, so Ben and I had to meet in the ward dining room. Any shift of our habits was jarring. We sat down on metal chairs at one of the round tables. On the wall was a framed print of two blooming apple trees.

We both sat there with the pad and pencil between us on the table, neither picking it up to begin, both looking at the poster.

"I've thought of writing about it," offered Ben.

"Today or other times?" I asked.

"Other times," he said.

I made no move. Nonchalantly, he slid the pad in front of him and began.

"Nature has much rain all over the colorful fields."

"Two blooming apple trees," I add.

Ben holds the pad up to his face, pondering, then writes, "A very large setting."

The Sun Rose Big and High
The Veil of Metaphor

Still a bit chilly, it's early spring in New York. But Dennis and I are south in Washington, D.C., for the day, and it's warm. We're on our way to meet with the National Endowment for the Humanities to raise money for the Poetry Project at Rosedale. We get in a taxi at the airport and drive by masses of flowering cherry trees; the air smells like heaven. A raucous song about love gone wrong is blaring from the radio. The windows are down.

"Have you ever been to the Vietnam Wall Memorial?" Dennis asks.

"No," I say. His floodgate opens. He tells me about the small town in West Virginia where he grew up. He tells about how he joined the Army during the Vietnam War. The memorial overwhelmed him—all those names, all that death, his history and the country's.

"I want to take you there."

There we are, out of the Rosedale context. There is loose sentimental music, sweet air wafting into the cab, and when he says "I want," I notice it.

Later that day, we are on a plane heading north to New York. Dennis is reading the paper, and I am looking out the window. We're above the clouds. The sun is gleaming. I take my book of John Donne poems from my purse and start to read. I come upon the poem "The Sun Rising."

"Hey Dennis, listen to this."

Busy old fool, unruly Sun
    Why dost thou thus
      Through windows and through curtains call on
      us?

"I just love those lines. Do you realize how much Ben and I write about the sun? It keeps coming up all the time. I wonder why. What do you think it stands for?"

We chat in an easy, rambling way, noticeably less intense than during our meetings at the hospital. I glance out the window at the sun and clouds and pretend to doze off. My eyes closed, I think how Dennis had said "I want" earlier in the day and let my head rest on his shoulder as if I were asleep. I catch myself and realize what I'm doing.

"Sorry," I say. "I was pretending to doze off so I could put my head on your shoulder, as if it's an accident."

"You don't have to pretend. Just rest your head there."

And so I do, gazing out the plane window at the unruly sun. For the moment, what seemed taboo is gone. Finally I doze off.

The sun, colors, stones, storms—these were the metaphors Ben and I used over and over in our poems. But the way he wrote about them changed. One reason our work could go as deep as it did without interpretation or explication is that we were drawn to many of the same metaphors.

On the ward, the patients' use of metaphor took on particular importance. Metaphor acted as a veil that protected their privacy. At the same time, however, it offered a means of honest expression. The patients' privacy was threatened when they watched TV in the ward living room while nurses observed them through a window. Their behavior and thoughts were probed, examined, and documented, whether they talked to themselves or played pool. These measures were taken to best understand and treat the patients, but the loss of privacy could harm their dignity. For example, whether a person showered or not, whether they smelled, became public information. When they wrote about what mattered to them from behind the veil of metaphor, their dignity was maintained.

It may be a monumental act to simply place a word on a page — this, I know from experience — so I encouraged patients like Ben, who wrote or spoke sparsely, to write anything. Whether their words were "good" poems, "bad" poems, or poems at all was irrelevant.

Ben mentioned the sun in nearly one out of four poems. By writing about the sun, he could indirectly express complicated ideas and feelings. Midway in our work, I started to register how often the sun appeared in our poems and that its qualities kept changing. I began to think that the sun stood for something else, although I had no idea what. Now I am puzzled that it took me so long to notice how often he wrote about the sun.

During our third meeting, Ben introduced the sun for the first time.

I'm a leaf (K)
I'm always in a good mood (B)
I move around with the wind (K)
I enjoy the sun (B)
The colors it makes in the sky (K)
everything's always fine with me (B)

If the sun was a symbol in this poem, there was nothing at the time that made me think so. There is very little to say about it. The sun was presented in a vague, general way. Although I started the poem by personifying a leaf — that is, *being* a leaf — I was not sure he went along with the idea of transformation, whether he was writing as a leaf or himself. Because his use of language was so bare and repetitive, any variation would have stood out, but none did. His lines mirrored his sparse speech: "Everything is fine," "Everything is well," "Everything is okay."

Many months later Ben introduced the sun again, and from then on, its qualities kept changing. Once, it seemed dependable: "The sun shines high above in the sky even though the weather is cold." Later: "The sun could be seen shining behind the mountain . . . for a far distance." Even if the sun was not completely visible, it existed. Whatever the sun stood for, it could be counted on.

Ben's father had a drinking problem and often arrived on the ward drunk. When asked about this, the father said it was not true. Ben denied it as well. Finally, as a matter of course, his father was required to take a Breathalyzer test before coming onto the ward. This setup worked until the day he returned Ben to the ward after a pass with whiskey on his breath, slurring his words.

There was a flurry on the ward about how to deal with this.

"Everything is okay," said Ben, when asked about it.

"I'll start," he said the next day when he sat down to write.

"The sun is glaring," he began.

Although Ben refused to discuss what had happened with staff members, he showed his dismay in his poem with the use of the word *glaring*. *Glaring* is far from *okay*. To write "the sun was glaring" was his opaque alternative to saying "everything is fine." Writing a poem, as opposed to speaking, made it possible for Ben to admit difficulty, masked though it was.

Several months after Ben and I had started to work together, Ben's psychiatrist found me in the nurses station. In a state of excitement he said, "We are finally beginning to exchange a few superficial sentences during our sessions! 'The day is cloudy,' Ben says. Then I say a sentence about the weather and wait. It has the same kind of stilted back-and-forth that happens when you first wrote with him!"

As we kept talking, we both started to wonder if the written dialogues were bridges to the spoken ones. Their exchanges had the same pattern as our poems. One would offer a simple sentence, then the other did.

About six months after that, Ben's psychiatrist told me that his uttered speech was becoming more complex, following by about three months the pattern of the evolving poems. After one of their simple dialogues, Ben surprised him with a complex comment.

"In poetry, we've written about everything. We've extinguished the topics."

I had already begun to see that Ben's predictable, monotonous writing was slowly developing into more complicated, expressive writing, within the framework of our simple poetic dialogue. When Ben's doctor told me this story, I wondered more about the parallel expansiveness that was happening in his speech.

Ben's comment provoked all kinds of questions in me. What about his word *extinguish*? Did he think he had killed something off by boldly calling the sun *glaring*? Had he said the unsayable? Had he said all he had to say about the sun, colors, stones?

Did Ben mean that we had extinguished life from the topics?

Ben began a sudden and remarkable streak of storytelling soon after his "extinguished the topics" comment. By now, he had built a hefty foundation of symbols. He seemed liberated. Maybe it was his deepening grasp of how to use metaphor to say what he couldn't otherwise say.

Ben was in his room, in bed, when I arrived on the ward for our meeting. A nurse told him I was there. Meanwhile, I had gone into the nurses station to talk to someone. Then I saw Ben standing at the porch door, looking around impatiently, as if he could barely wait to begin.

"Where is she?" he urgently asked a nurse.

I had never seen him impatient. I stepped out of the nurses station. Ben flew down the hall, knowing I was close behind, opened the door to the porch with a *whoosh*, and sat down. He abruptly picked up the pencil and started to write, dispensing with our usual habits. Ben began a full narrative with the sun and a snowfall.

It was evening the sun
was going down everything
became chilly (B) throughout
the long night (K)

there was quite a frost (B)
white ice coated each blade of grass (K)

the sky was very black

it snowed, all through the night (B)
a hush fell on the land (K)

It was quite some
cold weather that night (B)
and how it lasted (K)
Mornings light still
left it cold (B)

The story is simple. The sun disappears; it turns
cold, dark, and snowy. The sun reappears, but it re-
mains cold. That week, Ben's psychiatrist told me Ben
was talkative after the psychiatrist had missed a ses-
sion because of a snowstorm: Ben had wanted to know
about the driving conditions. The fact that Ben was
brought to speech by this suggested again that weather
stood for something important.

The staff noticed that Ben seemed very sensitive
to absence—his doctor's or mine. In fact, the hospi-

tal record emphasized the following "special attitude" for Ben: "Toward unacknowledged feelings of loss: in the absence of the therapist and the poet, their images should be evoked through mentioning them from time to time and reaffirming the anticipated dates of their return."

"Cold is a good subject," Ben exclaimed when our narrative poem was finished. I realized how hard it was for me to understand how cold his world was. And I didn't know whether he liked it or not. My mind wandered to facts I knew about Ben, about Ben and sex.

One time when he was a young teenager, his mother returned home from work to find him in a "compromising position" with a girl. A few years later, the same thing happened, only this time Ben was with his best male friend. After that, his friend was found dead, apparently from a drug overdose. Ben's extreme silence followed this friend's death. Were these things connected? Was sex too hot, too dangerous?

After Ben gave up on words, Ben's father took him on a trip to Seattle in an effort to help his son get over whatever was ailing him. He arranged to have Ben spend time with a prostitute in a motel near the airport.

"It wasn't pretty," Ben eventually told his therapist. Is that why cold was a good subject?

"Cold is a good subject," said Ben when we had five minutes left. He didn't want me to read our poem. I got fidgety, aware that Ben was altering our habits. Not knowing what to do in the remaining time, I asked if he wanted me to read a poem I had written about Iceland, a cold place.

No, he said and made no move to leave. He looked happy. He said nothing. As I relaxed, I thought that writing his evocative lines had made Ben feel good. We sat comfortable and wordless until our meeting ended.

Almost a year later, I walked onto the ward and saw Ben sitting on the sofa in front of the television with a young, pretty student nurse. She had long, straight dark hair and was animatedly talking to him. His posture was rigid. Hers wasn't. His eyes looked lively and were fixed on her. A flash of jealousy came over me. In that moment, I realized how much I treasured being one of the only people Ben seemed to care for.

That day, Ben began our poem, and his mixed feelings about the sun grew.

A magnificent orange glare
filled the afternoon (B)
one particular time (K)

There happened to be much shine and
brightness (B)
much gleam in the air (K)

It was just a

particularly cloudy day (B)
that happened to come along (K)

All the color
captures the imagination (B)

Ben handed me the pad after the last line and I read it out loud, as usual.

"I think the lines are about something else, they mean something else," he blurted out.

I was dumbfounded. It took a lot of control not to say, "What do you think they mean?" But that would have broken our unspoken deal—I was not to ask questions.

In the poem, Ben's elation burst with the prominent "magnificent"; its many syllables drew out its meaning. "Orange glare" showed up again, now modified by "magnificent." Beautiful as it was, the sun dominated the time and the sky. "Particularly cloudy day" conveyed difficulty, its monotonous cadence suggested weariness.

Then Ben mused—"All the color / captures the imagination." "Imagination"—a leap into what sounded like the alluring abstract. "Captures" suggested there was no escape from the tempting sun. The sun—what did it stand for? I thought of the student nurse. I thought of John Donne. I thought of shoulders, warmth, Dennis. The enclosed world Ben and I had worked in at the start was slowly becoming larger.

Analyzing the poems Ben and I wrote is a knotty task. The poet William Stafford wrote: "If you analyze [poetry] away, it's gone. It would be like boiling a watch to find out what makes it tick." Like Stafford, I would rather let poems and metaphors speak for themselves. But, as the anthropologist Clifford Geertz points out, in most societies people have a need to analyze art. He wrote, "Even the Australian aborigines . . . analyze their body designs and ground paintings into dozens of isolable and named formal elements." Many artists in our culture both deplore analysis and find themselves doing it. For a moment, Ben himself called attention to metaphor after a year and a half of work. "All the color captures the imagination."

A few months before Ben was to leave the hospital, I went on a weeklong trip to the Yucatan, where my husband and I prowled the Mayan ruins, swam a lot, and generally had a jolly time. The day I arrived back for my meeting with Ben, I was still daydreaming about the jungle I had just seen. We sat down in our chairs on the porch.

"Where were you?" he asked.

By then, his question, while surprising, was not a shock. He was speaking more and more.

As I told Ben where I had been, I took a few post-cards from my bag as a way to get the poems going. One postcard was a photograph of a boat in a harbor, nice and safe. Another was a bright semi-abstract painting by Kandinsky—a portrait of a girl with vague features, somewhat scary. Another was an antique postcard of a grove of banana trees, lush and phallic. The last was a photograph of stone ruins in the jungles of Mexico. I asked him to choose one for writing.

Ben never once chose an abstract picture for writing. Maybe abstraction left too much to the imagination for him. If he wrote from a picture of a boat, for instance, he could trust that he would stick to the subject of a boat.

This day, he took a long, silent while to decide. He picked up the card of the stone ruins. He looked at it. He looked at me. His face became quizzical, his brow furrowed. He said nothing. He asked nothing. He paused, looked back at the card, back at me, and began.

There are many indications of
the past all around (B)
in the shape of stones,
how they're piled upon one another (K)

There are usually ordinary indications
but sometimes it is indicated in
weather or other things (B)
hail pelting ancient stone walls (K)

things strike a unique picture (B)

Did Ben feel it was against his own moral code to express his feelings without the veil of metaphor? I remembered reading about cultures in which it is against peoples' moral code to directly show certain emotions. In an Egyptian community of Bedouins, for instance, the sadness of loss is aired through poetry. Women might sit together sewing a tent and spontaneously recite their own poems about their losses. But they would not dare speak about loss directly.

The mute heart of this work is metaphor. Metaphor allows poetry to get written. When Ben wrote, "things strike a unique picture," I think he was saying that certain images from the outside world, like the sun or stones or weather, impress themselves on individuals. What the sun means to each of us is unique. Why a stone strikes a unique picture in one person and a different one in another is inexplicable. But we each have particular images that attract us and correspond to something inside us. We can use them in poems to address and express our nearly inexpressible ideas and emotions.

Because so many of the same metaphors held sway for Ben and me, metaphor provided a welcome and essential distance, as well as a welcome connection. The mask of metaphor made it possible for us to get to know each other, rely and care for each other, and grow.

Because thinking about Ben in a romantic or sexual way felt taboo, I simply didn't. As our work evolved, I'd allow myself fleeting thoughts like *He is one gorgeous hunk*, but that was as far as my mind went. On the other hand, with Dennis, the taboos were looser. So I found myself writing a series of erotic poems packed with metaphor, with Dennis in mind. In this way I could consummate my attraction to him.

Metaphors are not just static images that correspond to particular emotions or events. They can seem as real as the boat Ben and I wrote about or the erotic scenes I created, so that after writing I felt I had been on a boat trip with Ben or in bed with Dennis. This realness makes it possible for metaphors to be manipulated to try new things, to take risks and change.

One day near the end of our work together, I made a radical suggestion to Ben. By then he had made so many alterations to our habits, I was starting to feel free to take the lead sometimes.

"Why don't we try this today. What about if I write a line, then you write a line, and then you just go on writing?"

I had not planned in advance to suggest this, but for sure it was on my mind to start having Ben write more on his own before he left the hospital.

Ben was quiet. He stared at each of our chairs, then out the window. He stared at the walls, then the door. Slow motion. He let out a large and loud sigh.

"Okay."

Both sun and moon (K)
They both glisten the sky
the moon is white but
the Sun is very bright

They are far apart in the sky

the suns fast traveling
sends it all over

the two contrast very much (B)

As Ben was writing, I sat on my chair watching him. His face looked tired and lost. He wrote. When he finished, he handed me the pad to read it. His eyes were resting on the tree's leaves blowing out the window.

Ben wrote about the relation between the sun and moon. After they each affected the sky, they became distinct—the moon "white," the sun "bright." Although different, rhyming connected them.

As I was reading the poem, I was taken by surprise because I thought he was writing about our connection. Was he the white moon, colorless and cool and I the warm and bright sun—or was it the opposite? When he said they are far apart in the sky, as well as making them physically distant on the page, was he speaking of our distance? When he wrote, "the two contrast very much," I wondered if he was saying we were distinct.

Today as I read this poem, I see that the sun and moon might have stood for other things. Often when I thought the sun stood for me, I felt I was standing in for someone or something else, that the metaphor's meaning was many steps removed. One time I may have stood for dependability, another time I may have stood for coldness or goodness or his father or freedom or his mother.

"*Our* poem is good," he said when he had finished, emphasizing *our*. "Now let's write a regular."

"Both Sun and Moon" was the only poem that Ben wrote nearly on his own. He chose not to write another again.

Pointing to the pad, he asked, "Is this different paper?"

"No," I said.

It was the same as every other white lined pad we had used from the beginning.

Together, we wrote another poem. Then Ben got up to leave, but instead of walking out the door, he stood there, looked at each chair, then out the window. Outside the wind was blowing the leaves.

The Subject Is Blizzards
Telling Stories

Weather is alluring. As if his life depended on it, Ben glued himself to the television screen to watch weather reports of impending hurricanes, Midwest flooding, the effects of drought.

Before I set out to work on this chapter early this morning, I went online to check the news and found that bad weather had overtaken our heartland last night. The following tornado report was plastered onto my screen.

Whole Neighborhoods Flattened; Dozens Dead, Hundreds Hurt

A cluster of tornadoes tore through Oklahoma last night wiping out neighborhoods and causing dozens of deaths. A massive twister with winds of 260 mph struck Oklahoma City.

The National Severe Storms Lab said the tornado may have been a mile wide at times.

Police combed through debris as darkness fell, searching for survivors. Crumpled cars littered two highways. Natural gas leaked from several locations. Power lines and piles of carpet were everywhere.

"It's gone," LeeAnn Richardson said as she looked toward where her home once stood.

"Oh my gosh," one woman said, "I could hear it getting closer, the house started shaking then the big rumble."

Power lines popped and debris flew as the twister moved along from Chickasha, and cut through the heavily populated metro area. Witnesses said the tornadoes sounded like freight trains.

"We could actually hear the train sound for a long time, then for about 30 seconds you hear the snapping and stuff blowing around," said a resident of Moore, Okla.

He ran into a basement with several neighbors, where they had to hold the door closed as the twister plowed over them.

"Whoa, Whoa, Jesus," Theresa Jones said.

"We called on His name and I felt his arms come around us and save us from that tornado."

A 13-year-old girl said she saw the bay windows in her house cave in and the tornado swirling inside the house.

"I was freaked out at that point. I've seen it on TV, I saw 'Twister' but seeing it with my own eyes, tearing up my own home . . . it is hard to explain."

"The devastation is beyond words," a KFOR-TV reporter said.

Join an online discussion.

In this new millennium, our culture is fraught with invitations to talk, particularly about our personal catastrophes. The last lines of this news report highlight our dilemma.

"The devastation is beyond words."

Join an online discussion.

How do people talk about catastrophe, which can't be put into words—words, those limited things.

Today, many years since Ben had become silent, *not talking* about what happens to you has no place. And silence? Unthinkable. But as the reporter said, some experiences are beyond words, and that will always be true for many humans.

Yesterday, a catalog from a press that publishes books about writing arrived in my mail. There have always been books about how to write your personal stories, but the number has mushroomed. Here are some of the titles: *Writing Articles from the Heart, How to Write & Sell Your Life Experiences, Writing from Personal Experience, How to Turn Your Life into Salable Prose.* Here is a description of a book about writing one's life stories.

> The author explains how to turn life events into vivid personal essays and riveting memoirs. His friendly instruction and stimulating exercises teach writers how to: open up memory, access emotion and discover compelling material, shape scenes from experience, as life events become plot lines, populate stories with the fascinating, silly and maddening "characters" that surround them—their family members and friends. From drawing a map of a remembered neighborhood, to yelling in public as a method of capturing passion on paper, the author offers innovative techniques.

Whether on daytime television or nighttime television, in a chat room, in a memoir, or a poem, the thing to do is tell your story. "If your poem's autobiographical, all the better!" a renowned poet once said to me. What about imagination? The notion that it's hard to tell your story, or that it takes a long time to want to, if ever, has no currency. Indirectly telling your story through metaphor is less valued than it ever was. Remaining mum on any subject, disastrous or not, is done with. Privacy is gone.

"The patient was an exceptionally poor historian," wrote the doctor who interviewed Ben when he first arrived at the hospital. The story of his life, according to his parents, was dramatic and chaotic, but Ben had nothing at all to say about it. For me, from the time I was a ten-year-old girl with polio until a few years after I worked with Ben, I rarely said a word about it. Because of our shared sense of paralysis, I think our work opened up the subject for me, and eventually it became a story I was able and even wanted to tell. The process took years.

It must have been important that Ben could tell a story, *some* story, *his* story, *his* way. Writing collaborative poems gave him the chance. For Ben, speaking directly about his personal history was out of the question. He barely spoke, and when he wrote his words were barren and colorless. When finally he did begin to tell stories in poems, they were not directly about his life, but they probably expressed what his life felt like.

Storms were the main subject of the stories Ben told through poetry. Repeatedly, he brought up weather — sunshine, fog, and blizzards. These elements became parts of the storm story, and I encouraged this. In other teaching settings, the direct autobiographical thread in poetry may be warranted, but on the psychiatric ward, where patients are continually asked to talk directly about their lives, the transformation of using metaphor is freeing. For someone like Ben, who renounced speaking about his life or emotions, the chance to change them into symbolic poems was crucial.

As Ben kept writing about a storm, his story became fuller and more touching, although it always remained in the realm of metaphor. When we began our work, his concept of metaphor was unformed and his lines lacked narrative elements. But as he began to manipulate the masks, the metaphors, he slowly started to combine elements of storytelling—time, place, mood, and beginnings, middles, and ends.

As he elaborated his story of the storm over the time we met, he spoke aloud more and more. On the occasions he wrote narrative poems, his speech and behavior were markedly expanded. It seemed that the more he wrote the story, the more he spoke out loud.

One day after a few months of work, Ben and I went to the porch to meet. The windows were open and it was cold.

"Are you cold?" I asked.

I surprised myself by my question, which seemed almost too casually personal at that early stage. I could have been talking to my sons.

"No, I'm okay." He paused and added, "Are you cold?" exactly mimicking my intonation. *Back and forth*, I thought, but *talking*, just like our poems.

He asked me to start our poem and make something

up. Because he was still so silent, his words and his wish amazed me and made me feel attached to him. I felt blank, strangely like Ben.

"It's hard to write out of the blue," I said, showing him that I, too, could feel undone and blank.

It was snowing out, so I wrote, "Out of the blue fell snow."

Out of the blue fell snow (K)
a cold wintery snow (B)
that was blinding (K)
there were blizzards everywhere (B)
white breezes, the noise of weather (K)
it was enormously chilly (B)
not enough clothes to go around,
people froze (K)
it was a cold season (B)

The poem tells a simple story of a snowstorm. The story does not unfold because there is no sequence of events. But Ben began to create a mood, an important element of narrative.

Until this poem, Ben had avoided using the past tense. I would use it and he would ignore it. The idea of history, the past, was absent; only the moment was expressed.

But here, when he followed suit with "there were blizzards everywhere," I was excited. Why did he choose to use the past tense? Before that, did his world only include the present moment? Had the past been too upsetting to mention?

Ben's past was full of pain and he was not going to talk about it. He had gone from being a productive, popular, active boy to a silent, isolated, violent young man. The afternoon his mother found Ben and his best friend having sex on the sofa was one incident in a long string of difficult times. After this friend suddenly died, Ben cut off all contact with friends and began to watch television constantly. He told his parents to tell friends who called that he was not home, so they finally stopped calling. By the time he was twenty-four, he was a silent, hospitalized patient. These facts about Ben's past don't reveal what it was like for him to live them. But his stories of the storms suggest what it might have been like.

My "not enough clothes to go around" directly mentioned people; then I say they froze. When Ben wrote, "it was a cold season," the mood became strained.

"Enough for this poem!" he blurted out.

His speech was so sparse and passive that his emphatic sentence surprised me, made me edgy.

Many months later, Dennis and I went out for Chinese food. I was surprised by a question he asked.

"Why do you feel identified with Ben?" Long pause.

"Can't think of anything—I'm not sure."

We slurped our hot-and-sour soup and got on to other things—hospital gossip, the fun of mowing and weeding.

"Are you sure?" Dennis repeated the question later as we were on to our fortune cookies. By then, I had started to think of the frozen cat my husband, Paul, and I had seen on our walk. I had begun to put together my own story with Ben's.

"I was about to bring this up again. You know that I had polio when I was little—did I ever mention that to you?"

"No. Was it bad? What happened? When was it?"

We left the restaurant quickly and went back to the hospital grounds. We walked to the formal gardens in the pitch dark. It was a mild evening in late spring.

As we walked up and down each row of perennial flowers—iris, lungwort, digitalis—I began my story.

"I was ten years old, paralyzed on the polio ward in Grasslands, a hospital pretty near here. I don't think it even exists anymore.

"I remember there was a long wall of windows I could see from my bed. I spent hours every day watching the prisoners from Sing Sing slowly walk by in the snow. Their mouths moved as they spoke, but I couldn't hear them. I remember wondering what they had done to be in jail.

"One day, my friends, other polio patients, and I were on stretchers and in wheelchairs listening to the radio when the newscaster announced that someone called Dr. Salk had discovered the polio vaccine. Some of us made jokes; I know I did. And some kids didn't say a word.

"When it was getting dark that night, I looked out

the window and saw my best friend, Patsy, who was not old enough to come to visit. She wore a shiny gray jacket and her hair was shiny black. Lightbulbs on the ward were low, and the room was dim. I remember how she pressed her face to the glass. I couldn't get near the window because I couldn't move. All we did was wave. I remember the quiet and I remember I couldn't move."

Dennis didn't say much or ask much. Our talk was like air seeping into a closed trunk full of god-knows-what. But now something was ajar. I remember feeling how tall and solid he was and drawn to tell him a little bit about when I was sick. *Trustworthy*—that's what Dennis was.

Moving his limbs with ease and pliability, Ben was walking down the hall to the porch when I arrived for our next meeting after our "Out of the Blue" poem. Watching him, I could see how he had once been an athlete. His normally rigid posture was relaxed.

"This is very interesting," he said when I handed him last week's poem.

It was hard to resist asking him how so. But from the start, I believed that if I were to ask him a question, he would take it as an invasion.

Without my asking if he wanted to start our poem, he picked up the pad to begin.

"The subject is blizzards," he announced with zest.

blizzards are tremendous (B)
moving from one place to another (K)
they freeze everything (B)
their winds batter (K)
unbelievable weather conditions (B)
for anywhere (K)
with everything frosted (B)

the blizzard caught a band of gypsies (K)
quickly they tried to leave it (B)
but the wind encircled them (K)
altogether quite cold (B)
wrapped in red woolen blankets (K)
much concern for the conditions (B)
much fear (K)

but nothing annoying happened (B)
the blizzard kept on (K)

No time, no place, no event—the poem begins with a general description of blizzards. But when Ben added "unbelievable weather conditions," I was startled. Instead of simply reporting on the qualities of blizzards, he reflected on them with the word *unbelievable*. His line was subjective, emphatic!

Because he was usually like a blank slate, I was used to imagining what he thought and felt, but now he was telling me. I needed time to adjust to Ben's newfound subjectivity in order to register how much of a person he really was.

When Ben wrote "everything frosted," I said I wanted the poem to end there. I may have needed time to adjust, but he didn't.

"Let's go on," he said and handed me the pad and pencil to continue.

For a split second, the room felt extremely tense, but Ben's enthusiasm was contagious.

I began a story with an event in the past, "The blizzard caught a band of gypsies."

With Ben's "quickly they tried to leave it," a story began to take hold. I added another event: "but the wind encircled them." When Ben wrote, "altogether quite cold," I couldn't tell if he was withdrawing. But I wrapped them in red wool blankets, offering relief and insulation to the people. In a flash, I thought of how my husband had given me a heavy red wool Hudson Bay blanket for my birthday early in our courtship and how much it meant to me. Symbolically, I wanted to do the same thing for Ben. Later, when I reread the poem, my line reminded me that Ben frequently slept in his clothes, and I wondered why.

The story took on dimension when Ben says the Gypsies are concerned and cold, telling how they felt both mentally and physically.

When I intensified his understated "concern" into "fear," I watched him read the page before adding his line. Suddenly, in response to reading my line, he dashed words onto the page like a speed demon, bringing the poem to a quick and contradictory conclusion: "but nothing annoying happened."

His line was mismatched in tone to the rest of the poem. I thought he wrote it in response to my use of "fear," which might have turned Ben away from the poem.

much concern for the conditions (B)
much fear (K)

but nothing annoying happened (B)
the blizzard kept on (K)

I had gone too far.

Around this time, Ben's therapist told me he was frustrated with the slowness of their work. Ben had told him a favorite nurse was leaving the ward. The therapist had asked how that was for him, and Ben said, "It's fine." As usual, he reacted to questions with silence or his pat phrase, "Everything's fine."

As my work with Ben progressed, my supervisory relationship with Dennis turned into a close friendship. By then he was feeling free to press me to think about my polio and Ben's silence. I told him about one day after I left the hospital and had gone home to recuperate, still paralyzed.

"I was in bed and I was watching the sun illuminate a ray of dust. The visiting nurse had just left. I was famished.

"I had to call downstairs to my mother to ask her to

bring me a snack. I remember thinking, 'If I ever walk again, I will not forget what it's like not to be able to walk, not to be able to run to the kitchen for something to eat, to have to ask someone for help.'

"Then, after I could walk I didn't really remember what it was like. I remembered words, but the words fell short. I was mad at words for not keeping the memory of paralysis exact.

"I think that my imperfect memory of paralysis, and also a frustration with the limits of language and of memory, is at the heart of my work with Ben."

As I was telling Dennis the story of my own illness more and more, I realized I still had a sense of immobility, although I had physically recovered. Ben seemed immobile too; only for him, it was mental. And what about Dennis—what made him so drawn to the work with Ben?

One afternoon on our way back to the hospital after a meeting in New York City, I asked him. We were zooming along the Hutchinson River Parkway. Saying it was stuffy, he opened the car windows.

Dennis had recently been divorced. I knew nothing about what had happened, except that it had been a long marriage that began when he was twenty. Dennis began to tell me about his two new kittens.

"Just as well that there's no wife around these days. I'm so done in by the time I get home from work, I have nothing to say. Touching and *no* talk—that's what I like about the cats."

"Touching and no talk—could be good," I teased.

By the time we were nearing the hospital grounds, Dennis had begun to tell me how when he was twelve years old, his father had a stroke and was unable to talk for the rest of his life. He had owned an insurance company in a small West Virginia town. His father had been astoundingly handsome—tall, sandy haired, athletic, outgoing. Dennis said he took after him, and I could see it. He had been a prize-winning dog trainer—sheepdogs. Before his stroke, his rough father had often beaten his three children. People said there was no relation between him before and him after.

All Dennis wanted was to be a good boy. He did contortions to behave properly. He said he never could decide which was worse—the beatings or the silence.

We pulled into the hospital parking lot. Neither of us budged. We sat in the car, windows wide open, continuing to talk. He asked something—I don't remember what—about my mother's death and Ben. I told him how in the three days before she died, I'd go to her hospital room and sit with her. She had an idea—she would talk and I would write down what she said.

"I don't like green," she had said. "We had a green rug. I didn't like the rug. Something seemed important about that green rug." She stressed *seemed*.

Stories kept coming. Back and forth. Dennis would tell one, then I'd tell one—all personal. But we each had appointments and had to get moving.

"Maybe we should go out for a drink after work," I said.

"Yeah—let's go back to that hamburger place in

Eastchester. I have a couple of private patients now. Why don't we meet in front of the main building at 6:30."

"The word *seems* is very important," Ben said after we finished the next poem that truly tells a story.

"I agree. *Seems* is different from *is*."

Not wanting to discourage his making these kind of acute observations out loud, I resisted saying more, but his insightful comment was thrilling. My cautiousness in speech was the same as in the writing. Let Ben take the lead. Don't scare him away from words by being too easy or quick with words myself. In my mind though, I agreed with Ben because *seems* reflects a personal, subjective point of view, which is critical to storytelling. Here is the poem.

One night the rain
completely chilled the weather (B)

its ceaseless noise pounded the roofs (K)

water filled the street (B)
rose up to the doorways (K)

clouds exploded causing more rain (B)

there was no sign of relief (K)

it was raining all over the sky

everything wet as the
temperature dropped very much (B)

floods, abominable cold, a plague (K)

the conditions seemed very harsh (B)

the villagers prayed (K)
eventually it stopped (B)

As the temperature falls, the story starts. This time, the storm caused a flood. Events took place when water filled the street. Something else happens when clouds exploded, causing more rain. As I read Ben's lines, I felt like I was reading a story unfolding.

When he handed me the pad, he stared at my face as I read how rain had chilled the weather, water had filled the street, and the clouds' explosion had caused more rain. I could feel Ben watching for my reaction, but his stare was nothing like his strange gaze from early in our work. Now it seemed he was reading my expression to try to discover what I thought of his line. This felt familiar from meetings with many other patients. My guess is that my face showed my excitement—all these things were happening.

Events dominated the poem. "The temperature dropped very much" is so different from Ben's earlier lines like "the temperature was cold." Now it felt like Ben was active as his verb became active. After my too strong "floods, abominable cold, a plague," he generalized from my specifics and turned the tone distant. Ben's conclusion, "eventually it stopped," was not incongruous, but it was abrupt. The storm stopped in this poem, but it reappeared in others.

The action in our poem was paralleled by a leap in Ben's speech the next time we met.

We sat down in our usual chairs and I put out some pieces of sea glass I had collected the weekend before, thinking we might use them for a poem. He barely glanced at them. He looked as if he was revving up to say something. Then finally, he looked right at me and said:

Ben: I was wondering what you would say about how I always write about the same subject.

    I began to answer, but he immediately interrupted.

Ben: I wanted to hear what you think about writing about a different subject.

    I began to speak, but he stopped me again.

KC: Do you want me to say something?

Ben: Yes.

KC: You've written so much about the weather this last year and I've thought that's okay. But now, if you want to write about something else, I imagine you will.

Ben: I'll be all right. I just thought you'd have something to say about it.

Ben picked up the pad and pencil. He took a long time before writing. I was shocked by our conversation in several respects. He wanted to know what I thought. He was introspective about his writing. All of this seemed monumental. And the sheer number of words we exchanged was as shocking as their content. Sometimes I wasn't sure what mattered more—Ben's increasing use of language or our increasing connection. To those of us who live in the talking world, this change may seem minuscule.

Finally, after what seemed like a lengthy conversation, Ben began to write.

There was a tremendous snow
which occurred out
over the middle of the ocean
It was rather cold and the
weather was very rough (B)
like a catastrophe (K)

It was dark raining
and the wind caused the snowy
weather to freeze (B)

This was no place for any man
or beast (K)

The sea water was so rough
that it was moving all about (B)
and no land anywhere around (K)

The rainy weather
caused very rough tides, (B)
high waves (K)

For the first time, Ben expansively began with a full five lines and a dramatic event in a specific location. A tremendous snow occurred in the middle of the ocean, and the weather was rough and cold. Although the poem has a full beginning, it has no middle and no end and no sequence of events, so it cannot be called a story. But the subject is the most impressive start to a story so far.

> A poem can be said to have two subjects, the initiating or triggering subject, which starts the poem or "causes" the poem to be written, and the real or generated subject, which the poem comes to say or mean, and which is generated or discovered in the poem during the writing. (Richard Hugo, "Writing off the Subject," *The Triggering Town*)

The poem's storm is strange. Was it raining or snowing? "Rough weather," "rough water," and "rough tides" brought seasickness to mind. My "catastrophe" played off Ben's "rough." My strong, short lines did not throw Ben's off-kilter. We were in tune with each other. Ben seemed supple in his bearing and in the structure of his lines. Consistently evocative, the language made sense without being logical. This was a poem.

"I really wanted to write a good one, since the poem was about the same subject," Ben said as we finished.

"You did," I said.

"Wanting to write a good one" might have come from Ben's valuing his writing and wanting his poem to be as good as it could be. Although he stuck with the subject of weather, he expanded the story.

Elsewhere, there were hints that people were beginning to matter to him. From the hospital record: "On a rare occasion recently Ben shared a spontaneous comment or two with the peer group. He told us what movie he and a peer planned to see on a pass and then reported back that they missed that movie and had to wait on line for another one. These small interchanges are experienced by the group as major breakthroughs in Ben's communication skills." Ben was entering the world of other people by speaking more.

"I'm very curious what particularly you think about this poem," said Ben after I read that poem aloud.

"It's exciting and contained," I said. *Just like you*, I thought.

"Yes, very contained," he said.

Now Ben asked me directly what I thought of our poem, instead of watching my face for a reaction. He seemed to grasp that he could use speech to help satisfy his curiosity. Words are just a tool. For so long, speaking had seemed to be an imposition on him, an invasion, even an insult to his privacy.

The movement of time is critical to any story. For

many months after we began to work together, Ben used verbs only in the present tense, then gradually he introduced other tenses. First he expanded from the present tense to the past, then after one year to the future. Using different tenses helped him tell a story.

Ben was becoming very interested in the subject of time. He wrote that time was always traveling, that time moved very fast, that time seemed complicated.

Time was paramount in the next poem. The tense was past, the setting was placed far back in time, and "Long Ago" was capitalized for emphasis.

Long Ago there was a dark night
with heavy snow
and much commotion and fuss all about (B)
and a wild wind (K)

people were all about but the snow caused
it to be very cold (B)
the people scurried around (K)

Long distance traveling was done
and it was very hard, (B) trying (K)

they wandered all around in
the freezing weather (B)
wondering where to go (K)

the snowy weather put everything
out of reach (B)
closed things in (K)

some people still wanted to
be out but couldn't (B)
they were snowed over
snowed in (K)

The night was very wild
and the snow was tremendous (B)

How could it happen
the ruthlessness of this wind (K)

It was all together a gala filled
evening (B)

"Long Ago" makes a great space in the past for the story to unfold and underscores the past. The story tells how a snowstorm and people are bound together. Now people are more prominent. The catastrophic mood of "There Was a Tremendous Snow" is here too, but with a major difference. At the end, the mood is annihilated. Had Ben become so expansive in telling his story that he needed to retreat? Three steps forward, one step back.

The heavy snow signals a storm. People in turmoil are implied with the commotion and fuss. When I read Ben's use of "people," I got excited, then more excited when he told what the people did and what it was like for them. "Long distance traveling was done and it was very hard." He added another event, portraying the people as lost—"they wandered all around in / the freezing weather." When he imagined what the people wished, Ben made a large leap—"some people still wanted to be out but couldn't." How people felt was on Ben's mind. They wanted something and couldn't have it.

The end of the story begins with "the night was very wild / and the snow was tremendous." The story begins in the first stanza, the next five stanzas comprise a hefty middle, and the setting is summarized in the end. My "How could it happen / the ruthlessness of this wind" took an outspoken look back at what has happened. Then Ben ended the poem, "It was altogether a gala filled / evening," obliterating its sense.

The more expressive Ben became, the stronger his retreat. Early on, when Ben ended "Blizzards Are Tremendous" with the line "nothing annoying happened," there was a similar jarring, denying effect. But in this case, the rest of the poem is clearer, more coherent, more complex, and more evocative.

Ben had done a lot of "long distance traveling." He was born in Israel and moved to the United States when he was five years old. He moved back to Israel for a year when he was thirteen. When Ben was in his early twenties and becoming more and more isolated, his father took him on that failed trip to the Northwest to visit a prostitute. On a long family car trip to Chicago, Ben started throwing candy at his older brother and then beat him.

As I looked at our poem that evening, I kept reading the line "Long distance traveling was done / and it was very hard." The next day, I had a strong wish to reread Ben's medical record, which included his personal history. I had not looked at it or thought of it for more than a year. That was my quirky way of immersing myself in our work—the poems on the page and the gradual growth of spoken language in our meetings. Rather than knowing the facts of his story, I concentrated on its feeling through his poetic lines.

After Ben had been at the hospital for over a year, Dennis wrote a report about him, parts of which follow.

A useful way to begin thinking about Ben was contained in the first line of the case record—"the patient was an exceptionally poor historian." Combining this fact with the patient's nearly psychotic level of denial and silence left us with very little beyond his daily behavior to construct a formulation, an approach or a treatment plan. We were in the position of archeologists trying to construct a civilization with only fragments and speculation, all of which was further complicated by the fact that the history that Ben did give was entirely different from the history everyone else gave about him. Finally, at the time I looked at the record, we had one year during which the staff participated in his history—one twenty-seventh of his life, so that we might have at least that percentage more sense of his situation.

In the protocol for the case conference prepared by his psychiatrist and members of the treatment team, I was able to identify several discordant statements. They began with the presenting problem in which Ben stated that his parents wanted him in the hospital but that he was fine. On the other hand, the parents' chief complaint was that he had been silent for five to six years. I wondered why this was their chief complaint, particularly given the patient's severe dysfunction, isolation, extreme suspiciousness, obsessive behaviors, refusal of food, and episodic violence. So there was a question about who the unreliable historian was, and who had what to deny and hide: there were radically different views concerning his drug abuse, the work history, and Ben's report that his mother gave birth to him after a pregnancy of three months. In addition to everything else, he thought he was premature!

After his birth, however, and up until about age thirteen, things are reported as pretty normal. There was some anxiety about starting school. In 1964 when Ben was five, the family changed countries (but we do not know why) and, with the exception of some understandable parental hyperbole, there were no problems during the later growing up years. The only discordant note in this story was the parents' report that Ben's brother "took care of him as a child and defended him to us." What did this mean? Against what in the parents did Ben have to be defended? And did this relate in any way to his reported need at age thirteen to defend himself with a pocket knife. Finally, did this raise questions about the history of the first thirteen years altogether?

I thought this line of inquiry was important somehow, because it was shortly after his brother's departure from home that the situation began to deteriorate. When he was thirteen, his father started drinking, and Ben started his so-called drug abuse.

My interview with Ben in which he said that his father never spoke of the war confirmed my suspicion

that Ben was not the only poor historian in the family.
It is, of course, one of the most commonly reported
phenomenons that survivors of the Holocaust have
done everything they could not to expose their chil-
dren to the horrors they endured — even to the point of
never mentioning anything about it to their children,
even when asked. The children, in a well-known and
well-described syndrome, begin to feel that there are
all kinds of unspeakable things that must be hidden,
denied, and feared. Wracked with the burden of their
parents' survivor guilt, these children also have mas-
sive separation anxiety. Ben's issues around separa-
tion seemed substantial, and he was quite clear that
although the hospital was okay, home was the only
place he wanted to be.

It gets even more complicated. What about Ben's
witnessing a suicide attempt in the unit bathroom and
not reporting it? What about refusing to eat bread
baked in an oven? And knowing what we now know
about the Nazi doctors, what about Ben's refusal of
treatment from the hospital's doctors? He told his
therapist that *treatment* is not even the right word.
This behavior and thinking could be circumstance,
it could be a paranoid solution, or could it be reen-
acting something important from mother or father's
unspoken and peripatetic Holocaust past?

I knew I was pushing the limited data pretty hard,
but it seemed possible that Ben was doing something
important for his family, especially his father. He and
father collude to erase and deface, to distort and deny
history, a history that appears unspeakable.

About five years after I reread Dennis's report and
five years after Ben and I wrote "Long Ago," I began to

have a surprising realization—*Oh, I wrote these poems too*. They also tell my story. My lines were not simply considered responses to his. If I exchange the word *snow* with the word *polio*, the poem could be about my own illness. Again, the subject of weather makes it possible to express the nearly inexpressible.

> the snowy weather put everything
> out of reach (B)
> closed things in (K)
> they were snowed over
> snowed in (K)

The night I got sick, it was dark and there was much commotion and fuss all about. The chaos made it feel like there was a wild wind. I was becoming paralyzed— "the snow [read *polio*] caused it to be very cold."

My fever was rising, my neck was getting stiffer, my legs felt rusty. Finally I couldn't move. Cautious footsteps came up the stairs. Two men rolled me onto a stretcher and took me outside. Neighbors on the street were silent, staring. They hoisted me into an ambulance. No sound, then sirens.

Next thing I knew, I was in Grasslands Hospital. When I woke up, I saw little metal crucifixes by my bed sent to me from students at the Catholic school near my house. I had no sense of time—no past, no future. Weeks passed.

A nurse was always sitting by my bed. Silently and meticulously, she did her nails. She'd file them, paint them red. I'd watch her remove the nail polish with a cotton ball. Then she'd paint them red again. These memories are wordless, vivid. Motionless, I would lie on my back, look at the lines and dots on the ceiling, and pretend they were animals moving. Sometimes I would try to turn over, but it was futile. I'd look back at the ceiling and again imagine animals on the move. Imagination was my close companion.

Three years later I was back at school and walking. But as a result of the polio, I had developed a curvature of the spine, the beginnings of a hunchback. I had to have an operation.

When I arrived at the hospital, I was taken to a room for four patients. Two were in plaster casts that went over their heads and down one leg to the knee. A hole for the face was cut from the plaster. A third girl was screaming that she would not have her hair cut.

My brown hair went halfway down my back. The hospital barber arrived in the room, and before I realized what was happening, he gave me a crew cut. Then I was taken to a large room with a wall of windows that looked out to the East River.

The day was extraordinarily sunny. There was a metal rack in the room. Spread-eagled, my arms were tied to two bars and my legs to two others. I was a thirteen-year-old girl with a crew cut and hunchback tied to a metal rack. Doctors took rolls of hot, wet plaster and wrapped it around me until I was covered, immobilized. As the plaster dried and hardened, it burned like fire.

Ben was a master of denial. His final line in "Long Ago" and in other poems denied the poem that unfolded before. Throughout his hospitalization, he maintained that he was there because his parents wanted him there—he was just fine. From the hospital record: "Most of the patient's unstructured time is spent in the bathroom, often he will be in there over ninety minutes. When asked by the staff why he was in there so long, he will deny that he was even there. When he was shown the 'SO board' (the written sheet that shows where each patient is at all times) to substantiate this, the patient states, 'It was someone else. I don't know why you staff write these things down.'"

Surely, Ben's denials somehow served him. Without his tight grip, fury might have flooded him. From the record: "One day in a peer meeting, Ben spontaneously began to discuss a situation where a co-patient was put into seclusion because of the co-patient's inability to control himself. His comments focused on this co-patient's need for containment and suggested a concern on his part that without containment he might get out of control."

Although negative consequences often come from denying reality, under some circumstances it is useful. When I was in the hospital paralyzed from polio, my parents urged me to talk to a psychiatrist, believing that I needed added support to survive the illness. Without knowing or caring why, I refused. Now I believe that by not speaking with a psychiatrist, I was preserving my optimism. Talk was no comfort to me. I knew I would walk again, a belief my doctors did not share. My denial of my dire situation allowed me not to feel defeated. I do not mean to make an analogy here; my situation and Ben's were vastly different. But my respect for denial comes from this experience and reminds me how important it sometimes can be and how attuned Ben and I were in this regard.

When I introduced a blizzard in our very first poem, "I Am a Stone," on the day Ben and I met, he made it clear that no matter how stormy the weather was, everything was fine.

(A stone) always comes through (B)
in any weather (K)
everything is always fine with it (B)
even in blizzards (K)
everything is always okay with a stone (B)

Something had stayed the same. "The gala filled evening" was a more forceful, more imaginative way of saying *no matter what, everything's fine*. But the way Ben wrote about the storm had changed. It's hard to imagine how torn Ben must have been between his wish to express and his wish to deny. At the very start, when he agreed to write poetry, he engaged himself in that battle. As Robert Browning wrote, "The story always old and always new."

The Sun Poured Yellow
Hints of Synthesis

"The weather's changed," says Ben. He has written a line, and instead of handing me the pad and pencil, he holds onto it. The room is silent as usual, which makes any sound particularly loud, like the wind at that moment. Waiting for him to hand me the pad, I'm confused.

"The real weather?" I ask.

In explanation I add, "We often write about the weather in our poems, that's why I asked."

Ben looks out the window, then directly at me with an expression that says, *Of course the real weather—are you some kind of goofball?*

Then in explanation he says, "It was warm, it got windy. I was outside, it got cold. I hope it gets warm again."

I laugh, then say, "Yeah, me too." Ben smiles, as if he, too, thinks it's funny.

It had taken so long for any exchange to be relaxed in any way, and this one took place near the end of our time together.

All this talking and writing about the weather—inner and outer. Later that day when I described the meeting to Dennis, *we* both laughed at how jerky one can become, finding meaning in everything. That day, the humor and absurdity of being plain old human overrode any built-in distinction of the workplace—patient, psychiatrist, poet.

In one of our last meetings, Ben listened to me read our poem. As he was listening, he looked out the window. The sun was out. He looked comfortable, his face looked soft, as if he were made from pliable material.

"It's nice to sit here and look at the light coming in the window," he said.

The first time Ben had begun to say sentences to me was four months after we had started our work.

Change came fast that day, and it was the only time in two years it did. We were writing "The Sun Poured Yellow," a poem that introduced and combined many basic elements of language for the first time: he used a personal pronoun for the first time, his vocabulary was less constricted, he introduced sound, and our lines spoke to each other. I was astonished that both his writing and speech were dramatically different on this particular, isolated day.

During the course of our long, slow expedition, the speed of change that early day gave me faith and patience. He said sentences, made suggestions, expressed opinions. Remembering how he wrote and how he talked that day helped me hold on to my attachment to him.

By the time Ben wrote the narrative poem "Long Ago" the following year, he was able to bring together various aspects of storytelling to write a moving story. It could not have been written without "The Sun Poured Yellow." By the time we wrote the earlier poem, I had begun to understand the unspoken ground rules of our work together: Ben generally was the one to initiate change in our pace and habits, and I was the one to maintain steadiness and constancy.

Bundled up in a big maroon woolen coat, I arrived for our meeting on that windy, snowy day carrying in the cold air with me. Driving to Rosedale had been good that day; I felt particularly free. An odd, unfamiliar freedom had begun to creep up on me since my mother's death the spring before. I was feeling easy and flexible. Everything was in motion.

I hadn't been thinking of Ben at all on my long drive south. I hardly knew him at that point, and although I was taken with him, his silence stumped me. I unlocked the door and walked into the warm ward. There was Ben, standing immobile in his usual spot by the nurses station. He was looking at the wall and smiling to himself. An odd thought passed through me, *Is he glued to the floor?* His arms were outstretched, a position he often held. Frozen—that's how he looked.

Ben seemed lifeless, and I remember how sad I turned the moment I laid eyes on him. I felt so free, and he looked so fixed. I had only known him for a short while, but already he had started to matter to me. We walked to the porch and had our usual exchange. First I handed him what we had written the week before, which he read to himself. He said nothing. Then I asked him if he wanted to keep the poems.

"No."

"Who should start the poem?" I asked.

Wordless, he motioned for me to start.

That day, I had decided not to bring in tangible objects for writing ideas. I wanted to try working at a new level of abstraction. So I brought in a few reproductions of paintings. Paintings were someone's interpretation of the world, rather than concrete pieces of the world like stones.

I placed the prints in a row on the floor for him to see. "Why don't you choose one you like," I said. He said nothing but picked up van Gogh's *Undergrowth*, which showed overgrown woods penetrated by some sunlight.

I picked up the pad and pencil. As usual, without saying anything more, I started the poem. I wrote a line and handed Ben the pad and pencil.

Land of Stone

The sun poured yellow into the woods (K)
they were hot all day (B)
they knew it would be hot tomorrow (K)
there was completely a lot of heat (B)
so that huge ferns thrived (K)

everything was very steady (B)
they found a shelter tree (K)
it was in the middle (B)
with umbrella-sized leaves (K)

there were many noises (B)
they began to sing (K)
everything was okay (B)
their song wove into the woodsounds (K)
most interesting singing (B)
pitch and tone the same (K)
far away noises could be
heard all over (B)

filtering through the ferns and leaves (K)

everything was smooth (B)

low and green (K)

many things at one time (B)

near and far away sounds (K)
distantly it could

be heard
interesting noises (B)

and close-up, their own (K)

When we finished, I was stunned by what had happened between us in our lines and our speech. Change had happened fast and on many fronts.

When I began the poem with the line "The sun poured yellow into the woods," all I was doing was describing the print. But when Ben added "they were hot all day," I thought he meant people were hot. And if that were the case, since there were no people in the print, *people* were Ben's invention.

Then he implied that something was affecting something else—the sun was making people hot. For the second time, Ben used the past tense. Before that, when I would introduce the past tense, he would ignore it and use the present. Here, Ben started to create a time frame.

The pace of change until this meeting had been exceedingly slow. So when Ben handed me the pad of paper with his first personal pronoun, use of the past tense, and introduction of heat, I wanted a line with shade to moderate what felt too fast-paced for me. Because our verbal and written exchanges had been so constricted, I must have expected and counted on constriction. Perhaps it freed me to pay intense attention to Ben's every move. The first time he broke the pattern, I got nervous.

Until this moment, I had not realized that the predictability of Ben's writing made me feel safe. It counteracted the discomfort I felt working with such a troubled and speechless person. Realizing this, I chose to go along with his heat and added the future tense. He continued by blasting the scene with more heat. By adding huge ferns, I articulated the idea that growth occurred in such a setting. When Ben wrote "everything was steady," he calmed the scene down.

Then, when he brought in sound—a new sense—I got excited by his word "noises" and moved ahead by bringing back people, who begin to sing.

Ben added, "everything was okay." In the past, that pat phrase had told me I had gone too far. Had I increased the intensity too much with the mention of singing? I did not think so, because of how expansive and active Ben had become. Because of the strong sense of synchrony, I took him at his word—things are going okay here.

Trying to knit together our ideas and keeping sound in the foreground, I wrote, "their song wove into the woodsounds."

Ben, whose sense of time was precise, was watching the clock. Always at this moment in our meetings, he finished one poem and wished to begin a second.

"Do you want to make this the turn of a long one and only write one today?" he said out loud.

I was arrested by the sound of Ben's voice. He said a whole sentence out loud. The words were not startling, but set against the backdrop of silence they sounded startling.

113

"Yes," I said.

That is when he added, "most interesting singing."
I added another fragment, "pitch and tone the same."

"Do you know what I mean?" I dared to ask.

"Yes," he said.

Suddenly our speech had loosened up. We were saying sentences back and forth to one another as we were handing the pad and pencil back and forth. Written and spoken language linked together during those thirty minutes.

I was amazed. I thought he must have keenly wanted to write a long poem if he was brought to speech by it.

Because Ben was moving so fast, I turned acutely cautious. As his pace of change quickened, I tried hard to stay put, so he could move forward if he wished. He had taught me this pacing by his ultra-sensitive reaction to any linguistic move I made.

As usual, when we finished, I read the poem out loud.

"It's *exactly* what's in the picture, *exactly* the same as the picture. It's a nice picture." As Ben said more sentences out loud, I remained stunned.

When I went down to Dennis's office for our meeting, I was still overwhelmed and became withdrawn. I needed to absorb what had happened privately before talking about it. I explained to Dennis the best I could that I wanted to wait until the next week to talk about the meeting with Ben. Whether he understood or not at the time, I don't know, but he took my need to heart.

We went to the cafeteria and had coffee and donuts instead.

A few years after Ben and I had finished our work, I was interested to see if the changes I believed had happened in his writing could be seen through graphs. I plotted graphs of when certain elements appeared in our poems—the sun, colors, curiosity, people, new senses, new verb tenses, emotion, narrative. I found that "The Sun Poured Yellow" was the only poem in which so many elements appeared together and many for the first or second time, underscoring my belief in the importance of that poem and that meeting. It was the day he began to say sentences. Surely, the writing and speaking were linked. The dialogue and harmony between us that showed that day in both the written and spoken lines were a foundation for the rest of our work. By the end, Ben could combine many features of language and poetry to move the reader.

In one of our last meetings, we were sitting in my office. There were a few opened books on the floor—I had been looking something up. My cheese sandwich and Coke were on my desk—I hadn't had lunch yet. Ben had tossed his jacket onto an extra chair. The room was relaxed. We wrote a poem, and this time Ben wanted to read it out loud himself.

"I like how it's coming all together—the sun, the mist, the heat, the water," he mused aloud when he finished.

115

His reflective comment was about synthesis, how our poem combined the elements of heat and water. I had noticed how our poem had synthesized elements of language and I said so. Now Ben and I were much less tense and careful together. Our words, spoken and written, and the atmosphere of the room had become nearly regular.

Aspects of my own life, which had seemed disconnected, began to come together during the time I knew Ben. Before, the story of my childhood illness had been completely shut away. I never thought about it, never mentioned it. Perhaps the synchrony of my early paralysis with Ben's mental paralysis, perhaps the way we approached it, helped open that chapter up. After Ben left the hospital, that story rose to the surface and got told.

It is hard to pinpoint the relation between the loss of my mother, an enticing distant character, and the appearance of Ben, another enticing distant character. Knowing Ben helped me come to grips with thorny aspects of my mother.

It is hard to fathom why things came together for Ben. Why he began to write poems and then began to speak aloud is hard to understand. But he did. Something had happened.

At the outset, why did Ben, Dennis, and I choose to make this long trek together? It was probably a mixture of simple things: I liked Ben, he liked me. I liked Dennis, he liked me. There were complex things, too, like Dennis's having had a violent, silent father. The three of us were drawn into the work because of hard old personal stories that touched on each others'. Our work paved the way for new ones.

Because Dennis was the supervising psychiatrist, Ben was the patient, and I was the poet-in-residence, we each had our distinct jobs to do. The larger, binding force, though, was the mesh of our unique human natures.

In his essay "Naming the Skin," the poet Donald Hall writes, "Of all the arts, poetry embodies best the whole of experience — because it combines in the same syllables abstract thought, historical allusion, dream, recollection, thigh and mouth." And for all three of us, poetry was the alchemist.

Stonework, Windwork, Waterwork
Final Meetings

It snowed all night long and all day yesterday. The deck must have fifteen inches of snow piled up. I've been working for hours this morning on Ben's story that happened so long ago. Time to take a break. The weather report says freezing rain is on its way. I better shovel the snow off the deck before it comes and ices everything up. I go to the closet, pull out Dennis's jacket, put it on. It's a tan windbreaker with a blue fuzzy lining and a torn right-sleeve cuff. Since Dennis is big and I am small, it's way oversized, but it's good being wrapped in it.

Dennis now runs a hospital in the Midwest. Long ago, the ties between us were strong, and they remain. Last fall, Dennis left his jacket in my car. I still have it and don't really plan on giving it back.

Long ago, Dennis bought a country house in a town near mine. I had recently stopped working at the hospital. But we rarely saw each other here in the country. Sometimes I wondered whether it was coincidence that he chose to buy a house so near me. Before moving west, he sold the house.

One chilly fall day a month before his house closing, we hiked a nearby mountain. The leaves were murderously red, still wet from a light rain. The woods were shining reflected light. As we tramped along, we were tongue-tied, but we covered miles of territory.

When we got back to the car, instead of parting we went to the town diner and got some good pie.

Afterward, we sat in the car.

"Okay—bye. I don't know what to say," I abruptly blurted out. "Good luck out there." Words seemed useless.

We leaned toward each other and kissed a long kiss with no reserve. Was it overdue? Was it taboo? Words seemed ridiculous. Dennis got out of the car and went to his, which was parked up the street. He forgot his jacket on my car's backseat.

Every few months now, we e-mail or chat on the phone. As for Ben, I don't know where he is or even if he's still alive. I've tried to find out to no avail.

Over time and slowly, Ben chose to raise his voice. As we alternated writing lines of poems for two years, our dialogue was the place where Ben's voice gradually became more resounding. We improvised our lines one to the other, never knowing where it would lead. I wrote a line, Ben wrote a line. Ben wrote a line, I wrote a line.

At first his silence secluded him in his own private world. Gradually, through writing poems and then speaking a bit, words no longer seemed like his enemies. Rather than invaders to his world, words helped him navigate back to the world of other people.

Weeks before the end of our work, Ben saw me reading a book as he walked into my office.

"Is that a special poetry book?" Ben asked.

This was the first time he acknowledged that other people besides us wrote poems, and he was curious about it. Finally the vacuum in which we worked was becoming less essential to him. Although this made me happy, I remember after his question thinking, *Oh, no, he's going to leave here.*

Toward the end, he followed a busy schedule of vocational rehabilitation and had an office job in town. Unaware of his job, I went to meet him on our usual day, but he was on his way out the door. He explained his situation and said he hoped we could figure out when to meet. I was surprised; this was the first meeting he had ever missed. As I suggested possible times, he seemed upset and said things like "that's the only time I get to go to the canteen for coffee and I have to do that." Finally, we agreed to meet the following Tuesday.

Tuesday arrived with no sign of Ben. It turned out that he had forgotten he was in a new group that helped patients adjust to leaving the hospital. We arranged to meet the next day at two o'clock. Wednesday came and the cleaning lady would not let us into our meeting room because she was washing the floor.

"Let's go upstairs," said Ben.

He no longer worried about meeting in a new place.

"This is a good room to write in; it's better," he said when he arrived there. Looking happy, he sat in the chair by the door and began to write. I saw that a button of his shirt was undone and noticed how nice his chest looked. I was in the chair with a large, open window behind me. The wind was blowing into the room. As he was writing, a thought went through my mind—*He's going to get up quickly, pick me up, and throw me out the window.* My own thought startled me. Did my reaction to his sexuality scare me and make me think he was dangerous? I calmed down as he was writing and considered whether there was any reason to be cautious with him at that moment. I decided that my surprising thought came from my own complex feelings about him and that my concern was unwarranted.

"After writing for a long time, words come differently," Ben said after we finished our first poem. By then, I had relaxed.

"For a change, why don't I read the poem?" he said when we finished the second one.

When he began to read, he enunciated each word softly.

Shortly before this, we had written a poem that began:

The voice (K)
It rises greatly (B)
swings over the room (K)
So loud that it causes a
great sound (B)

"For me myself, this was one of the most interesting topics we ever wrote about," Ben said with clarity and purposefulness when we were done. Both the poem and his comment flustered me. I looked right at him, and he looked back at me. I was speechless.

A bit before he left the hospital, Ben told me that his therapist had asked him what he would do without poetry.

"Poetry is a very big deal. But I don't need it," he said after a long pause.

What had his life been like in his years of silence before he started writing? What was it going to be like without writing? I told him that sometimes I work with people after they leave the hospital.

"All things have to end," he said.

Wondering what was going to happen to him when he left and feeling wistful myself, I picked up the pencil and began to write.

In a land of stone (K)
The sun would shine
bright there toward the ground (B)
connecting everything (K)

It indeed was a very bright place (B)
it was (K)

The sun would glare
all over the stone (B)
causing a heat (K)

The land seemed
colossal when it
was so sunny (B)
It did seem that way (K)

The stone was
unusually bright
too (B)
during what seemed like a fifth season (K)

After I added the last line, I handed Ben the page.
"The poem should be longer," he said, then reread
it. "I changed my mind. I think it should end with a
fifth season. The idea of a fifth season is so interest-
ing."

"Karen, I'll see you next week." He had never said
my name before. He got up to leave.

The following week we listened to music as we
wrote. Again, he asked me to start.

In fact there's a voice (K)
it relays and echoes
all around (B)

in the background, bell-sound (K)
The two together

produce sound everywhere (B)
The landscape is blanketed with their sound (K)

There is a lot of relay (B)
and boomerang (K)
The Sounds go far away (B)
they then resume (K)

Two weeks later, Ben told me that he might leave in two days or might stay another week. His discharge plans were unclear. He wanted to go home and work in his father's construction business, and his parents were willing to have him home. But the hospital staff felt it was important he live elsewhere, in a halfway house. This disagreement was still unresolved. I said to Ben that it was confusing not to know whether it would be our last meeting, then suggested we do what we always do—write. Ben seemed very calm. He sat in the chair and did not remove his light beige jacket. His shoulders were tense but not rigid. He looked at me directly but not intensely, as if he was beginning to move away. I looked at him and thought of his comment that all things must end. The room was still. It was fall. The tree outside the window had lost most of its leaves; we had seen many seasons through that glass. From that moment on, we both treated the meeting as if it were the last.

I put on some music, a duet from Bizet's opera *The Pearlfishers* that we had listened to once before, because the previous week he had said we should plan to listen to "something serious—opera." The tape was playing. We listened to the two voices singing to each other. The pad and pencil were on the ottoman between us. Neither of us made a move or said a word as we listened. Finally Ben picked up the pad and pencil and began to write.

> There are moments
> when everything goes
> slow (B)
> We have held on to that pace (K)
> huge spans of time occur (B)
> like bridges (K)
> when the sun sets it takes a long time (B)
> to disappear (K)
> There is a long time
> distance between each time (B)
> There is sun, there is stone, there is wind,
> there is sky (K)

When Ben mentioned the setting sun, I felt very sad. As soon as I wrote my line about disappearing, I was sorry. Was I too openly showing my own troubles with ending? But it was too late; he had the poem in his hand. When we finished the poem, the room was slow and sad. When I asked him if he wanted to read it out loud, he looked unhappy and said no. The music

continued and I didn't ask him if he wanted to begin
the next poem; it was obvious he didn't.

The duet of voices (K)
Much energy is felt (B)
back and forth (K)
There is a calm time
when there are many
things at one time, simultaneously (B)
in the midst of this long song (K)
differences occur
all over, (B) distinct notes (K)

Our time was nearly done, and neither of us moved
to leave.

"It's hard to think we won't be writing poems to-
gether anymore. It's been two years, and we've worked
hard," I said.

"Listening to music was good; it changed the sub-
jects of the poems," he said.

We only had a few minutes left.

I asked him if he wanted to write a third quick poem.
From his somber expression, he seemed to want to
write but didn't want to begin.

Stonework, windwork, waterwork (K)
there are many
large landmarks
all over (B)
to gaze on (K)

All the structures
are different (B)

I slowly read the poem out loud. He looked over all three.

"The word *duet* is a good word," said Ben.

I said that our poems had been like duets. He nodded yes. I wished him a good future and said that if he was at the hospital the next week, we would meet.

We started downstairs, he carrying the tape player. When we got to the locked ward door, Ben began to speak.

"It's been good writing poems with you. Poems have been good. We used words well. I kind of anticipated at the beginning that words would be the important part."

And we said good-bye. I went down to the staff meeting, and he went back to the ward.

Afterword
A Poet's Job on the Ward

The job I had before I went to Rosedale—teaching poetry writing to delinquent teenage girls in rural Massachusetts—came to an abrupt end in 1979. Two very large, rough female employees each took me by an arm, escorted me to my car, stood there while I got in, slammed the car door, and bid me adieu. "No poet's ever gonna set foot on this campus again. Get the hell outta here."

After working at Meadowview for a year, the inhumane treatment of the girls had come to an ugly, abusive head. I alerted Children's Protective Services and, of course, was immediately banished.

An earlier stint of teaching writing had sparked the evolution of my work. While teaching in Connecticut's Poets-in-the-Schools program in the late 1970s, I noticed that many students who had trouble in school liked to write poems. Teenage boys who caused chaos in the classroom and made fun of the "poetry lady" were curious when I showed them a pail of garbage and talked about how poems can be about anything— eggshells, one old shoe, last week's newspaper. Eventually, some of them turned seriously to writing. Perhaps these students were drawn to poetry because it contains a strong thread of rebellion, an aspect of poems I love and emphasized.

Later, when I began to work at Meadowview, the girls explained that they hated poetry because it had "big words" and was about "serious things like love." When I handed them onions and asked them to write a love poem to an onion, one girl said, "What do you want me to write 'I love you onion. You make me cry. You're so dirty. Your skin is so wrinkled.' Anyway, how can you love something dirty?" You can write things in poems that don't seem to make sense, I told her. Another girl suddenly said, "I love it. You can turn a toad into a train!" She had schizophrenia. When she talked to herself, she talked only about her illness. When she wrote, the world rather than her sickness became her subject. Her odd use of language was intriguing. "Write all the time—between chores, before dinner," I told her. "Make what you've written say exactly what you want it to say."

When I left Meadowview, I had a year's additional grant money from a foundation to continue teaching poetry writing but no place to do it. The grant was based on the democratic view that almost everyone gets satisfaction from self-expression, regardless of talent, whether they wish for it or not. So give people that chance. I visited an array of jails and hospitals in or near New York City with grant in hand and armed with the belief that poetry belongs in places it doesn't belong. Gun-shy from my school job, I searched for a humane setting to teach poetry writing, one where I would receive top-notch supervision.

When I visited Rosedale, it seemed like a fine place to explore my early ideas and questions. Here was a high-quality teaching hospital with a wide array of people with varying points of view. And I was not unfamiliar with hospitals. As a child with polio, I had been in and out of them, so I knew, apart from everything else, how isolating illness could be.

Rosedale's psychiatric residency program made for a lively academic climate, making it possible for me to learn about psychological illness. The wards offered opportunities for research and training, reflecting diverse views. Some stressed a pharmacological approach to mental illness; others emphasized psychotherapy or behavioral programs. One approach did not exclude the others; rather, it was a question of emphasis.

The people accepted for treatment at Rosedale had been hospitalized repeatedly and had shown they couldn't exist in the outside world. Most of what they did was explored as an expression of pathology. When the poet teaches writing on the ward, there is an opportunity for something else. The poet can read the patient's poem as a potential work of art that is effective or not, rather than as another expression of pathology. I was lucky to eventually find staff members who shared my view.

In time, as the Hospital Poet, I was conducting weekly poetry workshops and individual writing meetings with patients, meeting with clinicians, receiving supervision, offering writing workshops for the staff, and fully participating in case conferences. Eventually, we—I say *we*, because by then I was wholeheartedly a member of the staff—noticed significant changes in some of the patients. I began to work closely with a few clinicians to try to better understand what might be happening. The project grew. Workers from unrelated fields, poetry and medicine, embarked on a thoughtful collaboration. Fortunately, this was a time when wide-ranging exploration was possible in many psychiatric teaching hospitals.

People take turns talking. One speaks, then the other. If each person listens, hears, and responds to what the other has said, their speech is collaborative. When Ben and I met, we took turns writing, and in time our writing became more collaborative. In some ways, our written collaborations mirrored what happens when people speak, but a major difference was that we assumed we could remain silent. I made no push for us to talk.

People who have been through traumas sometimes stop speaking. After he was put away in St. Elizabeth's Hospital, Ezra Pound became silent. After the man who raped her was murdered, so did Maya Angelou. After Elie Wiesel survived Auschwitz, he took a vow of silence for ten years. What draws a silent person back into the world of words? How does a silent, or silenced, person bear witness to what has caused them to shut up?

People have countless ways to express themselves. Whether a person's life has been traumatic because of external events or because of inner turmoil, or whether a person's life has been relatively free of troubles, many of us eventually want to bear witness to our individual experience. People sing songs to bear witness, they reveal themselves over beers in bars, they tell their stories in support groups, they paint paintings to bear witness. What makes someone listen with attention to himself, claim his life as something worthy of disclosure?

The first nearly silent patient I wrote with once told me, "Ten years ago, I was half asleep all the time. The only thing that went in and the only thing that came out was poetry. My verbal skills were excellent, but I couldn't deal with people. The only contact I had was through writing."

Making contact with another person can entice someone to come forward and bear witness individually, and so can making art.

Artists work in isolation and they work together with other artists. Jazz relies on collaboration; players have to listen hard and spontaneously respond when they improvise. But most artists work individually on their creations, either in solitude or within a community. They work in their houses, in coffee shops, in studios — wherever they can be alone. Being part of a community also nourishes creative work. In the last century, the salons of Bloomsbury and cafés of Paris provided a place for artists to meet. Today, writers conferences spring up all over the map each summer for writers to affirm their citizenry. All over this country today, there are poetry slams. Poetry communities form in big cities and out-of-the-way towns, wherever a great, rich range of people come together to read and perform their poems, as well as to register their like or dislike of what they hear.

In some cultures, poets ordinarily compose poems together. In small villages in Morocco, for example, poets can go on for hours, as anthropologist Clifford Geertz notes in *Local Knowledge: Further Essays in Interpretative Anthropology*: "Poets sing alternately, sometimes the whole night long, as the crowd shouts its judgment, until one retires, bested by the other."

When I first came to the hospital, I mainly ran poetry workshops with small groups of patients. To begin, I would suggest that we all write a poem together, because that was a way people could be less afraid to write and share the burden of the page. People could also maintain a sense of distance by writing a group poem. Once I xeroxed Wallace Stevens's poem "Thirteen Ways of Looking at a Blackbird" and handed it

134

out to the people in the workshop. Each person read a stanza aloud in his or her own style—some slow, some fast, some staccato, some smooth. Because there were words people didn't know, one fellow looked them up in the dictionary and chimed in definitions as we continued reading. Someone asked what *inflection* meant. To illustrate, I made inflections with my voice. A patient began to make blackbird inflections with hers. I said that the poem regards blackbirds from different perspectives, that we were regarding the poem from different perspectives and voicing them with our own particular sounds. The room took on the sound of a low concert, each of us different instruments in the orchestra. Afterward, we wrote a group poem about birds.

Eventually, some of the students' desire to express themselves outweighed their desire for the comfort, fun, and stimulation of collaboration. So they wrote on their own.

Ray, a sad and articulate young man who had been active in the workshop for many months, became completely silent. He stopped eating and had to be fed intravenously. One day, after ten months of silence, I told him that the workshop was about to meet and that we would be listening to Scott Joplin piano rags before writing. With no words, he refused to join us.

Moments later, Ray walked into the room and began to mime playing the piano. I replied by doing the same. We were going to write a poem, I said. I would write a word, then he could say a word, which I would write down. After writing "piano," it was his turn. He sighed and appeared caught in the knowledge that saying the word *no* was saying a word, something he did not yet want to do. When I wrote "(sigh)," he laughed. Then he added a few words.

He rejoined the workshop and wrote poems with other patients, with me and on his own. Simultaneously, he started to speak again. Although it is impossible to know why, he was brought back into the community of words, in part while writing collaborative poems.

Many questions about collaboration arose when I wrote with patients. The first was always, Will the person meet with me or not? Most often, I chose to work with someone who was hesitant to speak. But I also taught patients who used words too easily, as if they did not weigh much. Patients might have met with me for a number of reasons. They may have liked me because I seemed like a regular person. Or they may have liked me because I seemed like an odd person. They thought poets have some glory or specialness that might rub off. They were writers or wanted to be writers, so they thought I might be able to teach them something. They may have felt pushed into it, or they didn't really want to meet with me but they were scared to refuse. Of course, not all patients agreed to meet with me. They might have refused because I seemed scary or because in the past writing had seemed too powerful and frightening. Or they thought they were too disabled to write. Maybe they valued poetry and felt that working on it in a psychiatric hospital was a violation. Or they were afraid of the pressure of work, or that meeting would be a waste of their time or my time.

With some patients, writing poems together seemed all wrong, not something to aspire to. And with some, writing collaboratively happened in roundabout ways. Beth, a highly educated woman in her thirties, came to the ward after she had been found psychotic and naked in the center of Stockholm. She spoke in a formal style that kept the staff and patients at bay. She walked around with a clipboard in hand and jotted down notes. Although Beth participated in the life of the ward, speaking freely at meetings and activities, her comments were extremely superficial. During our first meeting, she quizzed me about my thoughts on formal aspects of poetry, using words like *anapest, metonymy, hexameter.* At one point, I suggested that she try to be careless and thoughtless when she wrote in our meetings. She studiously jotted down my suggestion on her clipboard. Already, we were alerting each other about aspects of our own linguistic styles.

I gave her some scraps of wallpaper from an old house, suggesting that she write a list of words that the wallpaper evoked. When I asked her to choose the five most powerful words from the list, she said, "Should I choose them for their meaning?"

That question was her first show of unconventionality, because the conventional interpretation of my suggestion would have been to choose the words for their meaning. So, instructed by her question, I asked her to choose them for their sound. I read the words out loud, repeating them so she could take in their sound. When she wrote, her words had hints of expressiveness.

In later meetings, I sometimes gave her Rilke's poems in German, a language she did not know, and asked her to write her own poems based on the sound of Rilke's lines. Eventually, she wrote in her own dense, stark, evocative style. Words seemed to take on a new force for Beth. They seemed to be a tool rather than a barrier.

With some patients, finding a language to write together preceded finding their own style. With Beth, it happened the other way around. Nine months passed before we wrote a collaborative poem. Each was a production. We would add a few stanzas every week, editing as we went along. The common style we evolved was softer than her own—careful, precise, and very visual.

How do two people negotiate the ground rules of writing together? Who will initiate the poem? How will the poems be structured? Will each person add one line at a time, one word, or as much as they like? Does each person have the liberty to change the other's words?

When two people write together, how do they agree on a subject? In the early years, I relied on many types of stimuli, objects like stones or onions, tapes of music, or animal sounds. The idea was to offer the "third thing" on which the writers could concentrate. Finding a subject sometimes came from what had been written the week before. Or I might ask a patient to choose a line from last week's poem to get started. Sometimes the patient arrived with a subject already in mind.

An array of acrobatics takes place as the work of writing collaborative poems gradually progresses. Who takes the lead in a poem? How does a poem get grounded? Who lets it fly? The boat gets rocked; risks get taken that upset the balance. Who pushes the language boundaries in one way or another?

With great hesitation, Ben chose to raise his voice. As we alternated writing lines of poems for two years, our dialogue was the place where Ben's voice gradually became more resounding. We wrote our lines one to the other, never knowing where they would lead. I wrote a line, Ben wrote a line. Ben wrote a line, I wrote a line. Eventually, he began to speak out loud and returned to the talking world.

On the ward, my aim was to encourage patients to find their unique voice through writing and to help them determine whether they wanted to use it. It was always the patients' choice.

Even when I worked with severely ill patients, I always turned our work back to the writing. I might say, "Considering how awful you feel these days, how do you think we can move ahead on your writing during these rough times?" In other words, "The work of poetry writing goes on, simultaneous with your troubles. Keep this side of yourself alive in the midst of misery."

Although a talent for writing is unusual, a need for self-expression is nearly universal. The subject for poems is everywhere; they can be about anything. Whatever triggers a strong personal reaction is a potential subject. None is too small, too ordinary, too bizarre, or too daring. Whatever the subject, poetry requires genuineness. By genuine, I mean personally accurate. The poet tells his personal truth his own way through the poem's form and sound. If he is blessed with talent and is willing to work hard, the reader may see something startling that could not be communicated otherwise. Poems renew words so they ring out fresh from common usage. A poem can show a reader as well as the writer a small part of the world in a new way. The writer can be as surprised as Ben was with his own voice.

With Ben, it was only after he began to write with some expansiveness that the subject of poetry came up. By then each written or spoken word seemed less precious, thus less fragile. On the other hand, when a patient dashed off lots of lines, with no intention of working on the writing, I liked to be clear about the place of warm-up exercises, what makes poetry, and how the work of writing may transform an early draft into a poem. For people who use words in a facile way, as if they are weightless, I stressed their weight.

One reason I call what Ben and I wrote *poems* was

their high degree of authenticity. His genuineness helped his writing and helped me trust our work together. He seemed to stand behind any word he wrote or said, sparse though they were. There was neither pretense nor exaggeration nor puffed up sentimentality in his words. They all seemed heartfelt, and there were no false notes. Genuineness took a long time to surface with some patients, and of course with some it never did.

Poets at their most productive are freed by their flexible use of language. Psychiatric patients are often hampered by theirs. The wordplay used by some poets and patients often has different aims. Most poets hope to make contact through this unconventional use of language. But many patients' unusual language isolates them. The most extreme example is when a person makes up his or her own language. The result may be less communication, thus intensifying the need for unusual speech to express more isolation.

The poet in the psychiatric hospital has the job of not just stimulating writing but also teaching how to edit a poem until its qualities move readers to the place the writer wants them to be moved. Poems use language, sound, music, play, form, and meaning. The way these elements are synthesized affects the quality of the poem. When patients used language in an unusual way—punning, rhyming, making up words, condensing them—I tried to point out how this kind of language play could help or hinder the poem. A poem often combines unrelated images, other times called leaps or disjunctures.

I tried to teach a kind of revision, how to discard the leaps that obscure the poem and select those that enhance it. The depth and directness with which I talked about any of this depended entirely on the patient. Ben's relative speechlessness made me generally less direct with him. I highlighted how things can stand for other things in poems. Sometimes this use of metaphor came too easily, too naturally to patients, like when they made up their own language. Their words stood for things only they could fathom. Inventiveness, usually as asset, worked against them. When one patient wrote, "Louvre tumi sagili tumorlee," he left the rest of the world out. I told him that I had no idea what his line was about.

In the setting of the psychiatric hospital, where patients have many chances to talk about their feelings, I emphasized the process and craft of writing. Certainly poems must contain feelings, but they must also contain a host of other elements necessary to poetry. For example, when talking about a poem, I may have focused on how its musicality—its rhythm, pauses, stresses—affected the poem's meaning, rather than discussing the poem's meaning per se.

Chronic psychiatric patients lack self-esteem. When a patient has the unusual experience of being regarded as a student, a potential poet, rather than only a sick patient, her self-image may change. The unique experience of writing and working on a poem without exploring its personal meaning can be refreshing and nourishing. Many patients have abilities like humor and originality that are activated when writing poems. These qualities should not lie dormant during illness. When a patient's poem is read by others, one is no longer a solitary voice or as one patient said, "a small purple light going on and off in the snow that no one sees."

Once, a patient said to me, "When you write poetry you get to *use* your mind." His mind had seemed like his enemy because he often imagined he was being followed, mocked, or poisoned. When he wrote poems, he noticed that this same mind could serve him. Writing poems does not cure mental illness. But it can tap into and use the healthy, as well as the ill, parts of a person's mind.

For some people with schizophrenia, words take on the force of things rather than acting as symbols for things. Hearing the word *fire* might feel the same as fire. Words normally stand midway between the person and the thing, offering the safety of distance. If a person experiences the world with intense immediacy and expresses that vision in a poem, are they reporting, hallucinating, or imagining? As a teacher on the ward, it is important to keep these distinctions in mind. After writing what seemed like a wonderfully imaginative poem, a patient asked me, "Is it right?" He had wanted to write factually, realistically. And perhaps, for him, this would have been the best, most useful thing.

There are some dangers of being a poet working in a psychiatric hospital. One danger concerns what happens to the patients' poems once they are written. The poems are the patients' property.

This is a matter of dignity. They should not be handed over by the poetry teacher to the therapist to be used as takeoff points for therapy. In the same way, I would not suggest to a patient to use a dream told to his therapist as a jumping off point for writing a poem, enticing as that might be. On the other hand, if a patient wants to bring a poem to therapy, that's his business. Or the other way around: if a patient wants to bring a dream to a writing meeting, that's his prerogative. When we meet, I take care to encourage the person to use the dream as a point of departure for a poem, not for psychological exploration. Ben eventually began to initiate talk with his therapist about our meetings and, in a general way, our poems. And throughout, his psychiatrist and I talked in depth about our work with Ben, but the poems themselves were not shared.

Put simply, the psychotherapist has the job of guiding patients toward direct and conscious talk and awareness of their troubles, to help them gain mastery over their inner lives, with the goal of greater understanding and ability to go back out into the world and function. When a patient brings poems to therapy sessions, the psychotherapist has to be on guard not to be diverted or seduced by the poems. It can become a hindrance to their work. Merging therapy and poetry writing dilutes them both, although each is an expressive venture.

Another danger comes when the poet remains distant from the rest of the staff. The work done between patient and poet should not be sacred and separate from other work done on the ward. It is the poems that require protection, not information about the patient that might surface during the poetry meetings. By information, I mean aspects of a patient that might surface during our meetings but remain hidden elsewhere. If a person speaks gibberish on the ward but is coherent in his poems, this information should be shared. In planning a person's treatment or diagnosing their illness, this kind of information may be critical, and the poet has a responsibility to impart it.

As a worker on the psychiatric ward, it is a challenge to keep sometimes opposed aspects of a patient in mind. A patient may be an imaginative, hardworking writer who otherwise fights with everyone or sleeps. I may see her strengths, and the nurses may see her limitations. We each have to remember the side we don't see, whether we focus on it or not.

Another danger for poets is old as the hills. People tend to romanticize poets. The poet must shun being elevated as a romanticized truth teller, because being falsely elevated is really being diminished. Sentimentalizing the poet undercuts the potential value for interdisciplinary collaboration between artists and clinicians.

In the movie *'Round Midnight*, Dexter Gordon,

145

a jazz saxophonist, tells how different saxophonists play—how the swing bands play, how Lester Young plays like Debussy, how Charlie Parker plays—all different. "You just don't go out and pick a style off a tree one day. It's trees inside you growing naturally," he says. A poet and a clinician each provide growing conditions for trees, but the conditions are different.

Long ago, Oscar Wilde wrote a sentence that sounds archaic in today's self-revelatory culture. "A man is least himself when he speaks as himself. Give him a mask and he will speak the truth." Wilde's words are timeless, as true today as ever, because a human's wish for privacy is part of nature. Masks of metaphor made it possible for Ben and me to say things that were hard to say otherwise: stones, the sun, the wind and snow.

When the Poems Were Written

Beginning
11/85

I Am a Stone

I'm a Leaf

The Crockery Looks Very Old

Out of the Blue Fell Snow
Blizzards Are Tremendous

The Sun Poured Yellow

One Night the Rain

Imagining Colors
In a Room

It Was Evening

Middle
12/86

There Was a Tremendous Snow

Ordinary Indications

Towns Filled with Memories

Long Ago There Was a Dark Night

WHEN THE POEMS WERE WRITTEN

There Are Many Indications
A Magnificent Orange Glare

Both Sun and Moon
In Fact There's a Voice

In a Land of Stone
There Are Moments
The Duet of Voices
End Stonework, Windwork, Waterwork
12/87

The Poems

The Poems

A poem, being an instance of language, hence essentially dialogue, may be a letter in a bottle thrown out to sea with the—surely not always strong—hope that it may somehow wash up somewhere, perhaps on a shoreline of the heart. In this way too, poems are "en route": they are headed toward.
                                        Paul Celan, *Collected Prose*

Of the 179 poems Ben and I wrote, 22 are included here because of how they highlight linguistic change.

I Am a Stone

I am a stone
a stone is good
it sits on a field
it never worries
it never dreams
it always comes through
in any weather
everything is always fine with it
even in blizzards
everything is always okay with a stone

I'm a Leaf

I'm a leaf
I'm always in a good mood
I move around with the wind
I enjoy the sun
The colors it makes in the sky
everything's always fine with me

The Crockery Looks Very Old

The Crockery looks very old
from a bowl in someone's kitchen
it has a very smooth texture
smooth close up, smoothness
from a distance

it appears to be delicate

it's something to keep
I'll call it a "keeper"
it's a hot weather stone

Out of the Blue Fell Snow

Out of the blue fell snow
a cold wintery snow
that was blinding
there were blizzards everywhere
white breezes, the noise of weather
it was enormously chilly
not enough clothes to go around,
people froze
it was a cold season

Blizzards Are Tremendous

Blizzards are tremendous
moving from one place to another
they freeze everything
their winds batter
unbelievable weather conditions
for anywhere
with everything frosted

the blizzard caught a band of gypsies
quickly they tried to leave it
but the wind encircled them
altogether quite cold
wrapped in red woolen blankets
much concern for the conditions
much fear

but nothing annoying happened
the blizzard kept on

The Sun Poured Yellow

The sun poured yellow into the woods
they were hot all day
they knew it would be hot tomorrow
there was completely a lot of heat
so that huge ferns thrived

everything was very steady
they found a shelter tree
it was in the middle
with umbrella-sized leaves

there were many noises
they began to sing
everything was okay
their song wove into the woodsounds
most interesting singing
pitch and tone the same
far away noises could be
heard all over

filtering through the ferns and leaves

everything was smooth

low and green

many things at one time

near and far away sounds
distantly it could
be heard

interesting noises

and close-up, their own

One Night the Rain

One night the rain
completely chilled the weather

its ceaseless noise pounded the roofs

water filled the street
rose up to the doorways

clouds exploded causing more rain

there was no sign of relief

it was raining all over the sky
everything wet as the
temperature dropped very much

floods, abominable cold, a plague

the conditions seemed very harsh

the villagers prayed
eventually it stopped

Imagining Colors

Imagining colors
blue is very dark
when no light hits it

Yellow is very nice
on a cab, on a canvas

Red is Alarming
Red

These colors are always
around, they brighten up
everything and liven everything up

Up with color

Red goes very fast
it always goes fast
and is very lively

Zooming red

Things Always come alive
When Red is there

You can live in the color red

Colors can sometimes Be Very Dark

You wade through them
like through a swamp

They are always pleasant
they're okay

They sometimes fill the
Air with a bright glow
blueness

They always shine on
alarming everything

In a Room

In a room

colors are everywhere
on the four walls

the room is well decorated
proper

It is alarming being in the
room because it is so colorful
It has Much Gray

Each thing in the room
seems different
we reach for silence

It is a very good place
to be, to ruminate

It is Very Alive
within that space

And it looks Very good
in its formality

It is very well designed
its color, its shape

162

the different colors there
are very well chosen

the size of the room
in careful proportion

And so is everything in it
cautious in color, shape, and
silence

The room is Very exciting
within those steady walls

It Was Evening

It was evening the sun
was going down everything
became chilly throughout
the long night

there was quite a frost
white ice coated each blade of grass

the sky was very black

it snowed, all through the night
a hush fell on the land

It was quite some
cold weather that night
and how it lasted
Mornings light still
left it cold

There Was a Tremendous Snow

There was a tremendous snow
which occurred out
over the middle of the ocean
It was rather cold and the
weather was very rough
like a catastrophe

It was dark raining
and the wind caused the snowy
weather to freeze

This was no place for any man
or beast

The sea water was so rough
that it was moving all about
and no land anywhere around

The rainy weather
caused very rough tides,
high waves

Ordinary Indications

Ordinary indications–
coffee cups, curtains

What a setting had been
the kind of room to settle in

It was calm and peaceful
yet loud, a bunch of daisies
in a vase

Everything was going very fast
a strong wind blew the curtains

It was evening time and dark
there was much commotion and noise
time to turn on the lamps

There was a high mood of
orange in the room

Towns Filled with Memories

Towns filled with memories
These memories lasted long
their form changed

There was
a lot of water nearby
as if rivers could wash away
sounds

It was easy to remember
them, the towns being so big
The sky would often be red
unforgettable

Memories usually changed but
these didn't seem to
towns, sky, water hung on

They were as good in modern
days as they were in the past

Swift River, Red Sky, Bigness of Town

Long Ago There Was a Dark Night

Long Ago there was a dark night
with heavy snow
and much commotion and fuss all about
and a wild wind

people were all about but the snow caused
it to be very cold
the people scurried around

Long distance traveling was done
and it was very hard, trying

they wandered all around in
the freezing weather
wondering where to go

the snowy weather put everything
out of reach
closed things in

some people still wanted to
be out but couldn't
they were snowed over
snowed in

The night was very wild
and the snow was tremendous

How could it happen
the ruthlessness of this wind

It was all together a gala filled
evening

There Are Many Indications

There are many indications of
the past all around
in the shape of stones,
how they're piled upon one another

There are usually ordinary indications
but sometimes it is indicated in
weather or other things
hail pelting ancient stone walls

things strike a unique picture

A Magnificent Orange Glare

A magnificent orange glare
filled the afternoon
one particular time

There happened to be much shine and
                              brightness
much gleam in the air

It was just a
particularly cloudy day
that happened to come along

All the color
captures the imagination

Both Sun and Moon

Both sun and moon
They both glisten the sky
the moon is white but
the Sun is very bright

They are far apart in the sky

the suns fast traveling
sends it all over

the two contrast very much

In Fact There's a Voice

In fact there's a voice
it relays and echoes
all around
in the background, bell-sound
The two together
produce sound everywhere
The landscape is blanketed with their sound

There is a lot of relay
and boomerang
The Sounds go far away
they then resume

In a Land of Stone

In a land of stone
The sun would shine
bright there toward the ground
connecting everything
It indeed was a very bright place
it was

The sun would glare
all over the stone
causing a heat

The land seemed
colossal when it
was so sunny
It did seem that way

The stone was
unusually bright
too
during what seemed like a fifth season

There Are Moments

There are moments
when everything goes
slow
We have held on to that pace
huge spans of time occur
like bridges
when the sun sets it takes a long time
to disappear
There is a long time
distance between each time
There is sun, there is stone, there is wind,
there is sky

The Duet of Voices

The duet of voices
Much energy is felt
back and forth
There is a calm time
when there are many
things at one time, simultaneously
in the midst of this long song
differences occur
all over, distinct notes

Stonework, Windwork, Waterwork

Stonework, windwork, waterwork
there are many
large landmarks
all over
to gaze on
All the structures
are different